Divine Secrets of the Ta-Ta Sisterhood

Pledging the Pink Sorority

Joanna Chapman

Cosmic Casserole Press ◆ Concord, NC

Divine Secrets of the Ta-Ta Sisterhood: Pledging the Pink Sorority

© 2013 Joanna Chapman

Cosmic Casserole Press
366 George Liles Pkwy. PMB 156
Concord, NC 28027
http://www.cosmiccasserole.com
Cosmic Casserole Press...Serving up Honesty, Humor, and Hope

Some names and identifying details of people described in this book have been changed to protect their privacy. While this book is based upon my actual experiences, my memory is less than perfect. Any errors are unintentional. For narrative flow, some timeframes have been compressed and some conversations condensed.

The information in this book is intended to offer a personal recollection of breast cancer. This book is not intended to serve as any sort of medical advice. The author and publisher specifically disclaim any and all liability arising directly from information shared in this book. Consult a health care professional regarding your specific situation.

ISBN-13: 978-0-9890431-0-6

Library of Congress Control Number: 2013937370

Editing and interior design by Sarah E. Holroyd (http://sleepingcatbooks.com)

Cover design by Sarah Jensen (http://www.sarahlizjensen.com)

Printed in the U.S.A. (Lillington, NC)

Publisher's Cataloging-in-Publication data

Chapman, Joanna, 1962–
    Divine secrets of the ta-ta sisterhood : pledging the
pink sorority / Joanna Chapman.
      p. cm.
      LCCN 2013937370
      ISBN 978-0-9890431-0-6
      ISBN 978-0-9890431-1-3

1. Chapman, Joanna, 1962– 2. Breast—Cancer—Patients—
Biography. 3. Breast cancer patients' writings. I. Title.

RC280.B8C43 2013   362.19699'449'0092
                               QBI13-600065

"*Divine Secrets* chronicles the twists and turns of the sisterhood that no one asks to join. With humor and candor, Joanna provides an intimate look at the breast cancer journey, including helpful resources and side notes, just like a big sister would."
—Jennifer Johnson, co-author of *Nordies at Noon*, Young Survival Coalition

"Open and honest and written with a wonderfully light touch, *Divine Secrets* makes for some great company for breast cancer survivors at any point in the coping process."
—Mindy Greenstein, Ph.D., author of *The House on Crash Corner*, and breast cancer survivor

"The perfect antidote to the gloom and doom that comes with a cancer diagnosis. You will learn what you really need to know as she takes you through her experience with her eyes-wide-open yet light-hearted style. It is the *What to Expect When You Have Breast Cancer* guidebook any woman with a breast cancer diagnosis at any stage needs to read. What can you do for someone with breast cancer or someone who knows someone with breast cancer (i.e. pretty much everyone)? Buy this book!"
—Melissa Ackerman, MD, FACOG, ob/gyn, and breast cancer survivor

"Joanna is able to take a terrifying diagnosis and hold the reader's hand as she goes step-by-step through the emotions, the decision-making process, and the phases of treatment. The bite-sized Divine Secrets packed throughout offer truly priceless comfort and wonderful information. With snarky wit and sweet compassion, *Divine Secrets* is a must read for those diagnosed with breast cancer."
—Jennifer Smith, author of *Learning to Live Legendary* and *What You Might Not Know: My Life as a Stage IV Cancer Patient*

"Joanna takes her breast cancer sister by the hand and gently guides her through the journey to Cancerland with sincerity, genuine care, and a touch of much-needed humor. Her book offers practical tips and spot-on advice you would never have had without knowing someone who's already taken the trip. If you have a ticket on the Cancer Train, climb aboard but be sure to stash this book in your bags. Joanna reminds us no sister has to travel alone."
—Debbie Cantwell, founder of the Pink Daisy Project and breast cancer survivor

"*Divine Secrets of the Ta-Ta Sisterhood* keeps it REAL! You will find yourself laughing and crying at the same time. A must read for women in all stages of breast cancer."
—Mary H. Carson, RN, OCW

"This is just downright awesome. I love the humor…divine secrets are perfect!"
—Krysti Hughett, Young Survival Coalition

"*Housewives of Anywhere*, look out! There's nothing more real than hearing the words: *you have breast cancer.* A must to read and share!"
—Carole L. Sanek, RN, Director of *Breast Cancer Wellness* Ambassador Program

"Joanna Chapman's open and honest approach helps to answer key questions for a woman newly diagnosed with breast cancer. It's like going to a neighbor's house and talking it out over tea…it makes a scary situation less intimidating."
—Lisa Grey, author of the *Pink Kitchen* cookbook series

"Engaging writing style that absorbs the reader…Your book gave me a safe place to cry, to process feelings and give them voice…to reaffirm the strength of my human spirit."
—Betty Vitek, cancer survivor

"Keen insight into the life of a cancer patient. Hilarious, heartbreaking, insightful…with wicked wit and endearing charm and compassion."
—Gail C. Moore, cancer survivor

Dedication

To my sweet husband,
who definitely stood by me
"for better or worse;
in sickness and in health."

To my amazing mother,
who dropped everything to come
help our family
whenever we needed her.

To my circle of friends and family,
who delivered casseroles,
mailed care packages,
and kept me laughing
even during dark and scary times.

To all my pink sorority sisters,
near and far, optimistic or discouraged.
Sending you warm thoughts.
Still hoping and praying for a cure.

Table of Contents

Prologue:

Extradited to Cancerland

♡

Welcome to the Ta-Ta Sisterhood

Maybe you, or someone you love, just became a member of the "pink sorority" nobody wants to join. Perhaps you noticed a lump while showering or were called back after your mammogram. Maybe you have a strong family history of cancer and have been dreading the day you too might be diagnosed. Statistics say one out of every eight women will face breast cancer in her lifetime. Even if you never wrestle with the beast yourself, chances are someone you know and love will.

Regardless of circumstances, you are now a pledge of the Ta-Ta Sisterhood. Take my hand and I'll be your big sister, guiding you through the initiation rites of treatment and healing. Frankly, I'd rather have joined a sorority known for great keg parties. Let me turn the hospital sheet into a toga and spend my time in candlelit ceremonies, repeating obscure Latin mottoes. If I'm going to throw up, let it be caused by too much "trashcan punch" instead of chemo drugs.

But it is what it is: I'm a five-year survivor of breast cancer. Stick with me and I'll tell you the truth not everyone else will. Like, it's okay to hate all the Pepto-Bismol–pink knick-knacks. That treatment decisions can be perplexing. That your friends and family will need a "Stupid Pass" for their well-meaning but clueless comments.

I get annoyed with Pollyanna-ish survivors who say their cancer was a gift. If it's a gift, it's a tacky, passive-aggressive one, like Depends and Dentu-Creme wrapped up in sparkly black paper for a milestone birthday. I didn't need cancer to teach me a life lesson. Even so, the experience wasn't completely negative. Important relationships grew stronger. I stumbled over things to laugh about in the most unexpected places, my wacky and irreverent perspective carrying me through the toughest times.

While undergoing treatment, I'd get frustrated when I read a book or watched a movie with a surprising cancer plot twist. Never mind that Julia Roberts or Winona Ryder or whoever always looked lovely in their last moments, with suspiciously dewy complexions. Let me assure you that my story—blending elements of horror, suspense, and romance—has a happy ending, eventually.

I once was a fairly private person, but cancer has knocked down my emotional barriers. Maybe someday I'll be mortified about over-sharing, but if the disclosure of my breast cancer journey—and the unexpected secrets I've learned—can help another pink sorority gal, then it will be worthwhile. Therefore, I humbly offer you my story as a cosmic casserole, a cheesy comfort food, served up to you, my Ta-Ta Sisters, with honesty and humor, hoping it will make you laugh, cry, smile, and feel less alone.

I know we've been burned by unreliable memoirs in the past, so I promise I'll tell it to you straight, offered up raw and close to the bone, not deep-*Frey*-ed or sugar-sprinkled. But my mind is no steel trap; it's more like a stretchable aluminum Slinky. I probably won't get every detail right—maybe I *was* drinking a margarita rather than a piña colada when I had my epiphany about life's meaning on the top deck of a cruise ship. As a work of creative narrative nonfiction, the book's plot twists and turns are factual, though viewed through a subjective lens. At times my memory may be more impressionistic smudge than high-definition digital photo. But unlike the author who told readers he'd undergone a root canal without pain killers or anesthesia,

I won't claim to have performed my own mastectomy with a bottle of tequila and a Swiss Army knife.

If you're looking to me for medical advice, then you probably think Captain Kangaroo and Colonel Sanders work at the Pentagon. *Big mistake!* Consult your own physician for treatment recommendations. Also, while I've included the names of websites, books, small businesses, and nonprofits that I (or trusted friends) have found helpful, your mileage may vary.

As my Rock Star Surgeon likes to say, "You don't deal the cards—all you can do is play the hand you're dealt." Only a few years ago, I found myself at a high-stakes table, playing for my life. Take a seat, Ta-Ta Sisters, and I'll share a few of my trusty card tricks. *Game on.*

June 2013

Diagnosis:

Cancer is a Sneaky S.O.B.

1

Trouble in Paradise

July 2007

I lean back in the lounge chair, frozen strawberry daiquiri in hand. The ocean breeze at Hilton Head is refreshing, and I can hear the soothing sounds of the waves. Yet I'm anything but relaxed and content. Behind my dark sunglasses, I'm staring at other women's breasts more intently than a hormone-addled teenage boy.

I have breast cancer. Everything is different now.

Cancer can be one sneaky S.O.B. It's freaky how it can creep up on you without warning. There I was, a 45-year-old multitasking mom, feeling great, no worries...while underneath it all, malignant cells were stealthily multiplying. There was no lump, no pain, no outward sign to warn me that my life would change forever. If I hadn't gone for that annual routine mammogram—a few months overdue—the cancer would have continued to spread its tentacles, silent and menacing, for who knows how long.

Here I sit at this lovely beach resort, for what was *supposed* to be a relaxing, romantic, anniversary trip. Instead, I'm tormented by

Divine Secret: Everything can change in an instant.

All it takes is one phone call, one conversation, one appointment. Suddenly, life as you know it turns upside down.

anxious thoughts and tense muscles while questions multiply in my mind. I have a confirmed diagnosis of breast cancer and do not yet know my recommended treatment or prognosis.

Will I lose my hair? Will I lose my breasts? Will I lose my life?

Pieces of Me

My Pink Sisterhood story really started several weeks earlier, when our family was at Myrtle Beach, less than two hundred miles from Hilton Head, yet separated by a universe of differences. Hilton Head is an upscale oasis of chardonnay and polo shirts, live jazz and bike paths. Myrtle Beach is a mass-market nirvana of mini-golf parks and cheap souvenir shops selling hermit crabs, beer bongs, and Confederate flag bikinis. Instead of the ocean view of Hilton Head, our room at Myrtle Beach had overlooked a parking lot.

Nick, age 11, was playing in a basketball tournament at Myrtle, so we'd brought Alex, 14, and Larissa, 5, to turn it into a family vacation. In between games, we splashed in the hotel pool and hunted for seashells on the beach.

One afternoon, en route to yet another sweaty gym, I remembered to check my voicemail. After spending a dozen years as a stay-at-home mom, I'd recently gone back to work and started a grant-consulting business. In between messages left by friends and business prospects, there was a call from the breast imaging center asking me to come back for additional mammogram films.

Although I can be a hypochondriac and have several times googled myself into thinking I had some rare tropical disease,

I wasn't particularly worried. I'd been asked back for more mammogram films a few years ago and then received a follow-up call reassuring me that everything was fine. Frankly, the retakes just seemed like one more task to fit into my busy schedule.

∽

Now, a few days after our return from Myrtle Beach, I drive to a different imaging center, the one I've been told to visit. I walk in the door and start to feel a bit uneasy. There are two waiting areas: one for people undergoing routine screenings, the other for patients having diagnostic mammograms.

I look at patients in the diagnostic waiting room; all appear grim and anxious. Suddenly, I feel like I'm hyped up on multiple grande cups of espresso. I flip through a decorating magazine, but the pictures don't register.

Before long, a technician with a warm smile and floral lab coat ushers me into an exam room. I disrobe and wait for her knock on the door. She enters and positions me at the mammogram machine, tugging on my breast and pulling it into place. The cold glass plates squeeze like a vise. I wince, then grit my teeth and hold my breath as instructed while the machine hums.

The technician looks at the films.

"I'll be back in a little while," she says.

I sit there, a hospital gown covering my chest. A few long minutes tick by. I try to distract myself by observing the surroundings, but it's your typical exam room décor: industrial gray carpet, muted wallpaper, and nondescript chairs.

Surely they'll let me go home in a few minutes.

I check my watch again.

Then the technician returns, her smile still there but a bit dimmer.

"The doctor would like to do an ultrasound."

My ears ring with a nervous hum.

It's going to be okay, it's going to be okay.
I follow her to the room across the hall. I recline on the examining table; the paper crinkles. I look up, but unlike the dentist's office, there are no cheery pictures of puppies or rainbows tucked around the ceiling tiles. The technician dims the lights and pushes the equipment cart closer to the exam table. She squirts some gel on my skin, then takes the sonogram wand and begins rolling it across my right breast. I imagine what it must feel like to be a mouse pad. Minutes pass, as she keeps moving the sensor back and forth, up and down, frowning in concentration.

"Do you see anything suspicious?" I ask, hoping for reassurance.

"No, but let's see what the doctor says."

Soon the radiologist enters the room and introduces herself. She looks like a female version of the McDoctors on *Grey's Anatomy*: tall, slender, and gorgeous, her blonde hair pinned up in a chic chignon. The technician says she can't see anything, so the radiologist takes a look for herself. Though I'm supposed to stay still, I crane my neck in case I can see anything on the monitor. The screen looks to me like a clouded crystal ball, ominous and undecipherable.

I'm flooded with relief when she turns off the machine. *Everything must be okay if they can't see anything abnormal on ultrasound. Maybe it was just some weird shadow.* When the doctor and technician leave the room, I get dressed and wait for a nurse to dismiss me.

The radiologist returns, a sheet of paper in her hand.

"You need to have a stereotactic core-needle biopsy."

"I do?" I can't believe she's saying this. I stand there, as frozen as Bambi in a cluster of spotlights.

"We'll get you in as soon as possible, within the next few days. This type of biopsy is pretty sophisticated and only offered in one location, so you'll have to go to the Imaging Center downtown."

I nod, trying to disguise my disoriented emotions.

"With a stereotactic procedure, you'll be positioned face down on a special exam table with your breasts hanging through cut-outs."

Ugh, sounds freaky and scary.

"The biopsy is computer-assisted," she explains. "It uses mammogram-like digital views from different angles to target the suspicious area in question."

"What exactly are you seeing?" I can't understand how there could be something wrong without my knowing it.

She turns on the light box and points out a white speck on the mammogram film.

"See right here? This is a spiculated mass." She points out how rays, or stellates, emerge from the center. "Good thing you came in for a mammogram. It's located deep within your breast, so you wouldn't have felt anything during a self-exam until it was much bigger."

I stare at this evil spot, glowing like a splatter of luminous white paint.

"Maybe it's just a radial scar, a benign lesion that looks like cancer." She scrawls *radial scar?* across the top of the paper.

The radiologist escorts me to the checkout desk and shakes my hand goodbye.

"It's tiny," she says in a reassuring yet somber voice, patting my shoulder before walking away.

The clerks at the checkout desk look at my paperwork. One asks for my insurance card in a honey-toned voice dripping with sympathy. I leave with a biopsy appointment scheduled within a few days.

I walk to the parking lot, get into my minivan and let the news sink in. Everything seems surreal, as if I'm having a bad dream. No one in my family has ever had cancer. Surely I will be in the large majority of women who have breast biopsies and receive benign results.

But what if I'm not?

I think of Alex, Nick, and Larissa.

My eyes fill with tears imagining them growing up without me.

I think about Ryan, my husband of almost two decades, whose mother died of cancer when he was a college student, several years before we met. I can't bear to put him through something like that again.

I'm not sure exactly how long I sit in the parking lot, staring into space, before my cell phone rings. Ryan is calling to check in, just like he does at least once every day.

"Hi, honey," I chirp, struggling to keep any negative emotion out of my voice. I start chatting about all the activities our kids are signed up for that week. When he asks about my appointment, I try to sound unruffled.

"Just a tiny area they need to take a closer look at," I say. "I'm sure it's nothing. About ninety percent of biopsies turn out fine." Then, afraid my brave front will crumble, I change the subject.

On the drive home, I replay the appointment in my mind.

I'm healthy, I'm young. I don't feel a lump. I'm okay. I have to be okay.

Divine Secret: Girlfriend, don't put off that mammogram!

Getting your boobs squished like pancakes is nobody's idea of fun, but it might save your life. If you find a lump yourself, go see your doctor right away. Listen to your body and don't let anyone dismiss your concerns or tell you you're too young to have cancer.

∼

When I get home, I start googling "radial scar." I'm comforted that it sounds as if radial scars are harmless anomalies easily mistaken for invasive cancer, and that the only way to determine what is benign and what is not is to do a biopsy. This is reassuring—I tell myself the doctor is just being cautious and thorough. But when I search the Internet for "spiculated mass," my stomach twists like a vine. Every source says that a stellate lesion is highly suspicious of cancer.

Update: When to start routine screening mammograms?

In recent years, there's been debate about when to start routine screening mammograms. Some medical professionals say age 40, some say 50. (More of this topic later...) But one thing they all agree with is that screening should start early for women with a family history of breast cancer. Discuss your personal timetable for screening mammograms with your doctor. I'll concede that mammography is an imperfect screening tool, but it's the best option we have right now.

3

Hoping for a Diagnosis of Hypochondria

To avoid thinking about my upcoming biopsy, I reorganize the pantry, search for mates to unmatched socks, clean out the refrigerator, and chauffeur the kids to activities.

It doesn't work. I still worry.

The day before my appointment, I drive Nick to basketball camp. In the parking lot, I run into the mom of one of his friends. The boys have played on YMCA teams together and attended each other's birthday parties, so our families have become friendly. Basketball Mom is witty and funny, someone I always enjoy. And then I remember her husband is an oncologist!

"How are you?" she asks.

"Good," I reply, volleying back the socially acceptable answer. "How are you?"

We talk about our vacation plans for a few minutes. Then I try to nonchalantly ask her what type of cancer her husband treats.

"He sees a little bit of everything. But mostly breast cancer."

"That's great," I blurt out. "I'm getting a breast biopsy tomorrow." This is a pretty personal thing to share on impulse, but running into Basketball Mom seems like a fortuitous coincidence.

"Oh, no! I hope everything turns out okay."

"Me, too."

Basketball Mom scribbles down her husband's cell phone number on a scrap of paper and hands it to me.

"Please let us know if you need anything or just want to talk."

I thank her, reassured that I already know an oncologist, but hoping there won't be any reason to call.

～

The morning of my biopsy, I start feeling rattled. I see Hannah, an empathetic nurse and loyal friend, at preschool drop-off and ask her to join me for coffee. So we head to Starbucks, and after the barista hands us our mugs, we find a quiet table in the corner. I haven't told anyone except Ryan and Basketball Mom about the upcoming procedure, but now my emotions are bubbling over.

Over my skinny grande caramel macchiato, I tell her about the procedure scheduled for that afternoon.

"I'm sorry. I know it's scary. But I'm sure you'll be fine."

"Yeah, I'm hoping this is just another one of my infamous false alarms."

I share how I've worried about all sorts of diseases, even Sickle Cell and Tay-Sachs, both highly unlikely since I am both Caucasian and Presbyterian. I tell her about the first time I was called back for more mammogram films and a few health scares I've faced in the past.

"Before we adopted Larissa," I say, "China required parents to undergo extensive medical exams. After one fluke-y lab test, I was sent for a CT scan. Hypochondriac that I am, I got on the Internet and decided they were looking for cancer."

Hannah nods patiently.

"I started making a mental list of all the nice single women I knew—trying to figure out who'd be a good step-mom to my kids."

She laughs, but agrees she'd worry about her kids' futures, too. Wouldn't all mothers like to micromanage from beyond the grave?

Then I confide that while waiting for results, I spent an inordinate amount of time thinking about which photos—to be displayed at my memorial service—would not make me look seriously fat.

Hannah chokes on her skinny vanilla latte. "No one would ever accuse you of being shallow."

I reassure her, and myself, explaining that test results ruled out any serious medical issues.

My voice speeds up, wired by caffeine, as I tell her about my most recent scare. A few years ago, I started running a fever and a lymph node in my neck swelled up to the size of an acorn. Ear/Nose/Throat Doc had the hospital pathologist come to his office. A soft-spoken, bespectacled physician who'd trained at Johns Hopkins, Pathology Doc wheeled in a cart with microscopes and supplies. Though wincing from the sting of local anesthetic, I sat still as he plunged a needle into my neck. Then he retreated to the hallway to view the slides while Ryan and I waited.

About twenty minutes later, with a solemn demeanor, Pathology Doc walked back in the room with ENT Doc. "Looks to me like some sort of unusual infection or a low-grade lymphoma."

My stomach dropped. *Lymphoma? That's cancer!*

Ryan had a stunned expression, his complexion a sickly gray. We looked to ENT Doc for advice.

"You could have another biopsy to take out a larger sample," he explained. "Or undergo surgery to remove the suspicious node. Either way, we'll get results back in about a week."

I listened, feeling weirdly detached, like this was a scene I was watching unfold on TV.

"If you were my wife," ENT Doc said, "I'd want that node out." Ryan and I nodded in agreement.

ENT Doc went on to explain the details: a simple outpatient procedure, done under general anesthesia, with a quick recovery. He mentioned there'd be a scar, but in a few years it would be hidden by neck wrinkles.

My response was, "Gee, thanks, Doc, not only for telling me that I might have cancer, but also for pointing out that my looks are sliding downhill fast."

"But it turned out benign?" Hannah asks.

"Yeah, but it was a nerve-wracking wait. Then I bought some outrageously expensive moisturizer."

We laugh about how you can fret as much about the minor issues in life as the major ones.

I explain to Hannah that after the surgery was over, I was scheduled to go back in a week to discuss the results. I'd asked ENT Doc's office to please call ASAP if they found out the node was benign. I dashed to the phone each time it rang, hoping for good results. But the doctor's office never called.

"I was getting really scared," I say. "But Ryan convinced me to go to Atlanta for the weekend. Take the kids to a Braves game and keep my mind off things. But it didn't work. At the mall, I slipped away to browse through books about lymphoma."

While at the bookstore, I spotted Alice Sebold's new release, *The Lovely Bones*. Maybe it was a strange choice, written from the point of view of a girl who'd been brutally murdered, but I was struck by the urge to read it.

"The book was only out in hardback. I thought maybe I wouldn't be around long enough for the paperback. So I splurged."

We have another chuckle about my weird neurotic thoughts.

I tell her that, after waiting for days with no phone call from the doctor's office, I was glum, convinced ENT Doc had bad news to deliver in person.

"The nurse took us to wait in a conference room instead of an exam room," I say. "I assumed the worst."

Divine Secret: Take a deep breath and don't panic.

A biopsy is scary, but don't assume a worst-case scenario. Remember that most early-stage cancers respond well to treatment and do not spread or recur. Even in more advanced cases, new drugs may succeed in slowing progression, helping doctors and patients manage cancer like a chronic disease.

Finally, ENT Doc came in, but he didn't sit down.

"Your results were just faxed in. It's benign." He shook his head in disbelief. "This is great news. I'd expected a different result."

Ryan and I walked out of his office, giddy with relief and thankfulness. The sun shone brighter, the birds sang more beautifully, the flowers bloomed just for me. Life was good.

"See, you've been through this before," Hannah reassures me. "This will be just another false alarm. We'll be laughing over coffee next week."

Resource: Websites providing helpful information about breast cancer

- American Cancer Society: cancer.org
- Living Beyond Breast Cancer: lbbc.org
- National Cancer Institute: cancer.gov
- Susan G. Komen for the Cure: ww5.komen.org
- Young Survival Coalition: youngsurvival.org
- Imaginis—The Women's Health & Wellness Resource Network: imaginis.com

Drill, Baby, Drill

Early that afternoon, I drive downtown for my breast biopsy at the specialized radiology location. After checking in, I take a seat in the reception area and smile wanly at two middle-aged women in colorful dresses sitting across from me, both holding tissues and dabbing their eyes. I'm not sure which one of them is the patient because they both look worried and upset.

I've always been very independent, so I hadn't asked my husband or a close friend to accompany me. Instead, book lover that I am, I bring reading material. (There's nothing worse than to be stuck in a doctor's office with only tattered waiting room copies of *Sports Illustrated for Kids* and *Diabetic Living*.) Glancing down at my lap, I realize I've brought two paperback books and two magazines. *What was I thinking? That I was going to be stuck in the waiting room for 30 hours rather than 30 minutes?*

After I reread the first page of a book for the third time, a tall brunette nurse calls my name. She escorts me to a room, asks some questions, and then leaves so I can change into a gown. I've only spent a few minutes with her, but there's something brusque and unpleasant about her manner. Shouldn't "niceness" and "caring disposition" be *prerequisites* for becoming a nurse? In the same way that elementary school teachers should actually *like* children?

The nurse returns, instructing me to recline on the exam table. She wants to do a sonogram to locate the suspicious mass prior to the biopsy. I'm flat on my back as she rolls the wand around on the upper outer quadrant of my right breast, peering at the monitor.

It makes me sad that this situation is so different from the last time I'd had extensive ultrasounds. When I was pregnant with Nick, it had taken several appointments until my obstetrician could get a clear view of whether he was a boy or a girl.

The nurse keeps looking for the suspicious area, to no avail.

"They couldn't find anything the last time with the sonogram," I tell her. "Both the ultrasound tech and the radiologist searched for a long time."

"I'll find it."

"It's a spiculated mass," I say. "Only visible on the mammogram films."

"Oh, are you a medical professional?" she asks, arching her thin eyebrows.

"Uh, no."

She's thinking I'm just one more hypochondriac with Internet access.

Snippy Nurse slides the ultrasound wand to the inner upper quadrant and begins moving it around.

"That's not where they were looking before."

No response. I stare at the ceiling, wishing I were any place else.

"Found it!" Her voice sounds almost gleeful. She writes some comments on her clipboard and leaves the exam room.

I sit up, feeling forlorn and anxious. I should have brought Ryan to hold my hand or a good friend who'd whisper a few snarky jokes to break the tension.

Snippy Nurse returns a few minutes later, accompanied by the radiologist. He's an older man with kind eyes and a reassuring manner.

"Let's take a look." He gestures for me to lie down on the exam table. After glancing at the nurse's clipboard, he, too, examines my breast with the sonogram. He moves the wand to the inner quadrant, closer to my cleavage than my armpit.

"That's not where the other radiologist looked for it."

"Yes, dear, but breast tissue is soft, not rigid," he reassures me. "You are lying down, in a much different position than when you had the mammogram."

Okay, sounds reasonable. After all, this guy does ultrasounds and biopsies every day.

The doctor injects my breast with numbing medication, waiting a few minutes for it to take effect. Then, we walk down the hall to the stereotactic biopsy area.

Wish I hadn't come alone; I could use a good luck hug. Right about now.

In addition to Kindly Doctor and Snippy Nurse, there are several more nurses and radiology technicians waiting to assist. I climb on the table and one of the women helps position my body correctly. I hear a whirring noise as the table is raised and tilted. The platform is elevated, sort of like the hydraulic jack used to rotate your car's tires. I end up in a most undignified position, my butt in the air and my breasts hanging down through two holes in the exam table.

Suddenly, my middle-aged breasts are attracting more attention than those belonging to a Hooters waitress. The room is filled with tension, but it's not the sexual vibes created by young women in orange hot pants and tiny risqué t-shirts. Instead, it's the nerve-rattling tension you get when multiple medical professionals in white coats are examining you closely, not saying a word.

I feel vulnerable and exposed. I'll pass up an 80% off clearance sale if I have to use a communal dressing room, like at *Loehmann's*. But here I am, topless in front of half a dozen strangers.

A different nurse instructs me to hold very still as my right breast is compressed by panes of an X-ray device. Several technicians stare at computer monitors. They're taking images from different angles so that the computer can calculate exactly where to collect the tissue sample. They reposition my breast against the glass multiple times to get the data they need. Kindly Doctor wipes my skin with sterilizing solution and injects more lidocaine to numb the area. It stings a little, like a bug bite.

I turn my head to see the computer monitors, but since I took off my glasses, everything in the room looks fuzzy. The nurses remind me to stay very still. I squint to see their faces and listen to their voices, trying to decipher any clues.

After the additional numbing medication kicks in, the radiologist pierces my breast with a rotating needle that whirs like a power drill, vacuuming out tissue samples. I feel a little pressure but no significant pain. He tells me they'll leave a staple behind to mark the area biopsied.

A staple? Like from OfficeMax?

As he labels the specimen tube, I steal a quick glance at the tiny chunks of tissue inside, wondering if anyone can tell without a microscope whether they are benign or malignant. I climb off the exam table and am escorted to another room, where a typical mammogram machine is located.

"I need to take a few more pictures," Snippy Nurse says. I comply, as my breast is squashed once again. Feeling drained, I want to get out of the building as quickly as possible.

Suddenly sympathetic, the nurse examines my hole-punch divot and warns me that I'll be bruised. She fetches an ice pack, then presses it against my breast.

I flinch from the cold.

"I need to put firm pressure here. I know it's tender, but the ice will help. I really don't want you to feel sore and uncomfortable over the next day or two."

Now—after the scary drilling needle part is over—she decides to act nice? What's up with that?

Snippy Nurse goes over the post-biopsy instruction list, reminding me to take it easy and not pick up anything heavy. I wonder why she's had such a personality change. *Perhaps she's bipolar or battling major PMS mood swings?* Sorry, it's too little, too late to change my impression. I return to the dressing area and put on my bra and blouse. I hold my books and magazines under my left arm as the nurse escorts me to the exit door.

I stop at the central desk, where Kindly Doctor and several technicians are chatting.

"Excuse me," I say. "When should I expect results?"

"It usually takes several business days," a blonde woman replies. "You'll hear back from your doctor."

I wonder which doctor she means. I haven't contacted my primary care doc, and since I've only seen my gynecologist for one or two annual pap smears, I barely know him either.

Kindly Doctor explains that most people prefer to get results from their personal physician. But I assure him I just want to learn something as soon as possible. The anxiety of waiting seems more than I can bear.

"My husband and I are going out of town in a few days," I explain. "I was hoping to hear before we leave."

"It's Thursday afternoon," he says. "Your results may not be back until the middle of next week."

The blonde lady suggests that I call tomorrow, late Friday afternoon, to find out the time frame of when to expect an answer from the pathology lab.

I thank them and trudge out to the multi-level parking garage. *Surely mine will be just one more of the high percentage of breast biopsies that turn out benign.* Once I get the "all-clear," then Ryan and I can relax at Hilton Head. I try to shake off the fear of the day's experience and think about our trip. I imagine myself sprawled in a lounge chair, lulled to sleep by the ocean sounds. Sipping frozen cocktails at

Divine Secret: Take someone with you to critical appointments.

No matter how strong or independent you are, invite a friend or relative along to offer support, take notes, ask questions, give you a hug, or hand you a tissue.

the poolside bar, dining at restaurants providing neither crayons nor kiddy menus. Without the children, Ryan and I can completely relax and sleep in. We will not have to apply sunscreen to multiple squirming bodies, count heads in the waves, or play pirate-themed mini-golf.

Surely this is just another false alarm.

Patience is Not My Virtue

The lyrics crooned by Tom Petty and the Heartbreakers are indeed correct. Waiting *is* the hardest part.

I call the imaging center the following morning even though I know it's too early to hope for any information. I call again late Friday afternoon, asking the nurse when they expect to hear from the lab.

"Actually, Ms. Chapman, your pathology report just came back."

"Already?" I'd anticipated they'd tell me to call on Monday or Tuesday. *But now they can tell me everything is fine; Ryan and I can have a stress-free vacation!* "Then, I'd, uh, like to know the results."

"We usually send the results to your doctor. Then the doctor will contact you."

It's almost 5 p.m. His office is closed for the weekend. "I know it's not what you usually do, but I'd like to know what the report says."

"You're sure?"

"Yes." *Arrrgh, why do medical professionals always act like they are guarding classified state secrets?*

"Okay," she sighs. "I'll let you speak with the doctor."

I take a deep breath while she hands the phone to the

radiologist on duty, a faceless, unfamiliar voice. Someone I've never met, not the physician who did my biopsy.

"You'd like to hear your results right now?" Random Radiologist asks. His tone is neutral, giving nothing away. I swear, professional poker players must teach bluffing techniques to medical interns and nursing students.

"Yes."

"It's positive."

I'm silent, confused for a brief second. *Positive means good, right?*

Alas, not in the medical profession.

"It's positive for cancer."

"Oh."

"I'm sorry. You'll need to see a surgeon. And I recommend that you get a breast MRI." He says a few more things but the words scramble in my brain.

Dizzy and stunned, I put down the phone. *I have cancer. This can't be happening!*

I head directly for the study and call my husband at work.

"Uh, I got my results," I blurt out. "It's cancer."

"You're kidding."

"No, I'm afraid not." The sound of my own voice is distorted, all breathy and strangled.

He's silent, struggling to process the news.

"Ryan?"

"I'm coming home," he says. "I'll be there as soon as I can."

I've read enough about breast cancer to know that there is much I don't know, an entire vocabulary of terms I don't yet understand. My mind reels with questions, but there's no one to ask. I feel like I've parachuted into rugged, foreign terrain in the dark of night with neither compass nor flashlight.

How am I supposed to get a surgeon? Or that MRI he mentioned? It's the start of the weekend, so I can't even talk to my primary care physician until Monday morning. Nevertheless, I call his office and leave a message with the answering service, asking for the first available appointment.

I glance out the window and see the boys riding their bikes. I can hear Larissa in the living room, singing along to the *Dora the Explorer* theme song. All of them blissfully unaware that our family life is about to implode.

Then I remember my conversation with Basketball Mom.

Her husband, Nick's former coach, is an oncologist!

Digging in my purse, I find the scrap of paper with his phone number. I leave a voicemail, explaining that I've just received news of a malignant biopsy. In the past, I've steered away from using the professional services of friends and neighbors, not wanting to complicate things. But this time the stakes are much higher, so I'll take full advantage of our cordial relationship.

My mind races with all sorts of questions.

How bad is my cancer?

Where should I go for treatment?

Will I need chemotherapy?

Am I going to die?

Friendly Oncologist calls back within minutes.

"I know this isn't the news you wanted, but we'll get you through this," he assures me. "It sounds like what you have is probably early-stage cancer, usually very treatable."

"The radiologist who read my diagnostic mammogram said it looked tiny."

"That's good."

He describes how cancer staging is done by tumor size, spread, and aggressiveness, and outlines possible treatment scenarios. He explains that I'll be juggling appointments with a number of specialists—surgeons, radiologists, oncologists— over the next few months.

As I'm jotting down notes, Ryan walks in, dismayed that I'm tied up on the phone. I tell him I'm talking to Friendly Oncologist. Listening to my side of the conversation, he sinks into a chair.

"Call me anytime while you get this all figured out," the doctor says. "I want to help however possible. I'll be out of town next week, but will have my cell."

"Thank you so, so much! I appreciate you answering my questions."

Before we end the conversation, he gives me information about some of the surgeons and oncologists he knows or has heard positive things about and promises to

Divine Secret: Get potentially bad news in person.

If you have a serious disease, you want that information to come from a trusted health care provider who has reserved time to answer your questions and explain what happens next. Ask a friend or family member to come along and take notes, because you won't absorb everything.

check back in a few days to see how I'm doing. I put down the phone and study my husband's face, crinkled with worry.

"Wow, I didn't expect this," he says, enveloping me in a hug. "It was hard to keep it together at the office."

I cringe with regret. Maybe it wasn't the best way to break the news, but I was disoriented, confused, and overwhelmed.

Update: Nurse navigators to the rescue!

In years past, it was not uncommon for a woman to be told she had breast cancer, advised to find a breast surgeon, then left to figure out things on her own. Now there's great news: by 2015, every accredited cancer center must offer patient-navigation services. Nurse navigators can help patients make informed decisions, answer questions, provide emotional support, set up referral appointments, etc. Make the nurse navigator your new BFF!

Does an Apple a Day Keep the Doctor Away?

I spend the weekend alternating between dread and disbelief. To my knowledge, there's no history of cancer in my family. The closest we came is my maternal great-grandmother who had a mastectomy back in the early 1970s. But that was before mammograms and breast MRIs, so who knows if she even had cancer? Maybe it was just a benign cyst. I'm anxious for Monday morning to arrive so I can talk to my doctor.

Picking up the phone, I call Mom. I hadn't told her about the suspicious mammogram or biopsy, so I know she'll be shocked. I hate the thought of telling her.

Glancing out the window, I can see my sons shooting basketballs in the neighbor's driveway.

"Hey, Mom," I say when she picks up.

She asks about the kids and how summer is going. We chat for a few minutes.

I summon my nerve and break the news. "Mom, there was a problem with my mammogram. I had to get a biopsy."

"Don't worry," she replies. "Most of those biopsies turn out fine."

I brace myself, trying to keep my voice steady. "I've already gotten the results back. And I *do* have breast cancer."

I hear her gasp. Then silence as the news sinks in. "Oh, I'm so sorry," she replies, her voice thick and strangely pitched.

I know I've ambushed her with this news. I may be 45 years old, with three kids of my own, but I'm still her child. I can only imagine how devastated I'd feel if Alex, Nick, or Larissa had a serious illness.

"Do you need me? I can be there in just a little while." Retired, my folks live in the mountains, about two hours away.

"Not now. But definitely later." I'm glad she's close by, not halfway across the country. I have a feeling it's going to be a bumpy ride.

"Let me know what you need. Anything."

"I will." Suddenly, I hear Larissa singing the *Barney* theme song in her room upstairs, the sound piercing my heart.

"Mom, we haven't told the kids yet. I don't want to scare them." I take a deep breath. "I don't know what to say."

"What have your doctors told you?"

"I don't know much at this point." I keep my voice calm but know she hears the strain. "We're hopeful it's early-stage, but don't know anything for certain." As I summarize my conversation with our neighborly oncologist, she agrees his involvement will be a great benefit.

"Sweetheart," she implores, "let me help however I can. And you know Pop will do whatever he can for you."

When my mom and stepfather retired, they left Arizona and moved much closer. I was already grown, married, and expecting Alex, before Pop became a part of our lives. Though he's technically my stepfather, he's become my virtual dad, sharing a love of travel, a sturdy sense of humor, and a knack for dreaming up entrepreneurial ideas.

"I'll stay at your house as long as you need," she adds.

I feel so thankful that she's there for me. We weren't always close while I was growing up. Over the years, we've become more relaxed and less guarded, more tolerant of our differences and accepting of each other's quirks. Like the fact that she irons everything, even dish towels, while I rely on wrinkle spray. Or that she's constantly reorganizing, while I'm happy to close

closet doors without stuff tumbling out. But despite our differences, we appreciate each other, and I know she'll be there to
help me every step of the way.

~

On Monday morning I get a call from my official primary care
physician's office. They've scheduled an appointment for that
afternoon. Though I've been going to this medical office for the
past eight years, it's rare that I actually see the doctor. With a rep-
utation of being brilliant, he's in high demand. However, he has a
staff of four physician assistants, who are nice and give you plenty
of time to ask questions. I've never minded seeing one of the PAs
on the rare occasions I go in for something like a sinus infection.
But when it comes to cancer, I want to talk to the top dog.

My appointment time arrives, and I'm sitting on the exam
table, reviewing the questions written on my notepad. After
taking my temperature, a nurse checks my blood pressure and
pulse. A few minutes later, the doctor enters the room looking a
bit like a mad scientist, with a mass of wavy black hair, a goatee,
and thick Coke-bottle glasses.

He's very smart, so I'm sure he'll guide me in the right
direction, giving me the answers I need. So confident of this,
I'd urged Ryan to stay at his office, insisting I'd be fine at the
appointment on my own.

"I see you have breast cancer," he says, glancing up from
his clipboard. His tone is nonchalant, as if I'm there for some
pedestrian problem like heartburn or toenail fungus.

"Yes," I answer. "I found out late Friday afternoon. When I
called to check the status, they told me the results were back
from the pathology lab."

"Our office received a fax this morning."

"Well, I asked them to tell me. And then the radiologist
advised me to get a breast MRI."

The doctor crosses his arms and furrows his brow. "That's not
standard protocol."

What's not standard protocol? Does he mean the breast MRI? Or is he ticked off that the imaging center told me the biopsy results instead of allowing him to disclose it?

"I don't usually order MRIs for my breast cancer patients."

I'm temporarily speechless, reeling as if I'd recently touched a light socket rather than a finger pulse oximeter. This is the doctor who ordered a dizzying array of tests for me in the past, all of which turned up nothing. *And now, when I have a confirmed diagnosis of cancer, he's balking at tests that could help me?* My eyes begin to water, but I blink back tears.

"Can you recommend a breast surgeon?"

"Any of the surgeons here would be fine."

His response makes me uncomfortable because he's affiliated with a community hospital offering (at that time) only general surgeons. Nothing against the physicians or facilities here; they were great when Alex had his tonsils removed and when Nick had a ruptured eardrum repaired. But I'm dealing with cancer; I want an oncology surgeon—not someone who spends most of his or her time removing appendixes and gallbladders.

"Shouldn't I go to one of the National Cancer Institutes?" There are several highly acclaimed universities with medical schools and cutting-edge research facilities within a day's drive. "Or at least one of the large cancer centers downtown?"

"Why would you want to do that?" he asks, looking bemused.

I feel a flash of anger, shocked by his condescension. "Because I'm 45 and breast cancer tends to be more aggressive in younger women."

Okay, I admit "younger" is a somewhat relative term. But since most breast cancers are found in women in their 60s and 70s, I'm considered young from a diagnostic perspective.

"I have a good friend in New York. He's the best there is in treating breast cancer. I can send you to him if really necessary."

Well, maybe his friend is the top expert, but he's a thousand miles away. Not really practical for my situation. This appointment is not going the way I expected. Tears start rolling down my cheeks.

I glance at the nurse. She gives me a sympathetic look.

I've never cared much about a doctor's bedside manner, always choosing a physician considered genius-smart but not necessarily friendly and personable. I'm not the type who sends photo Christmas cards of the kids to the obstetrician who delivered them. Plus, I've always thought it better to keep some relationships strictly professional.

I pick up my notebook and pen, ready to start asking questions.

Doctor Doofus sighs and rolls his eyes.

I dissolve into a full-blown *uuuuuuuugly* cry. I don't care if a doctor doesn't spend much time with me if I have strep throat or pink eye or an ingrown toenail. *But, damn it, I have cancer!* Maybe my questions will put him behind schedule, but with a life-threatening disease I deserve a little more time than someone complaining about arthritis or an overactive bladder.

I'm gulping for air, struggling to speak. My eyes and nose are streaming like Niagara Falls.

"Never mind," I snuffle, gathering my belongings.

"I want to help you," says Doctor Doofus, in the same tone one would use with a recalcitrant child. "You need someone to coordinate your medical treatment."

"Thanks, but no thanks," I choke out, then flee the exam room.

Storming through the crowded waiting room, I cause a stir, unable to hold back tears of frustration. Patients look at me with a mix of curiosity and sympathy, trying to decide whether I just heard bad news or if I'm crazy.

In the parking lot, I take refuge in my minivan, overcome by great sobbing gulps. I feel alone and scared.

What do I do?

Who can help me?

I don't know where to turn. I'd been counting so much on this appointment, thinking I'd leave with answers and a clear battle plan. I glance in the rearview mirror. My face is tomato-red, my cheeks tear-stained. I've got to find another doctor, someone both smart *and* nice who won't be annoyed with my questions.

Where should I go?

I can't go home. I can't stop crying.

I've got to get a grip on this and calm down. I don't want to upset Ryan and the kids. They've seen me cry before, but never like this, unable to string together a few words without great heaving gulps.

Then suddenly I think of a solution. I'll go see my gynecologist! He has an easy-going, empathetic demeanor. I've only seen him a handful of times, but he's used to dealing with hyper-emotional pregnant and menopausal women every day, so he won't be rattled by my tears. Maybe he can help me calm down and figure out what to do next.

I call his office and explain my situation. The nurse encourages me to come in. The doctor will work me into his afternoon schedule. She says they got a fax from the breast imaging center that morning, since their office had originally ordered my routine annual mammogram. She tells me they'd already tried to call my home number.

~

By the time I get to the gynecologist's office, I've regained some composure, but my red, glistening eyes and puffy face give away my emotional fragility. The waiting room is filled with expectant moms reading parenting magazines. Before I can sit down, a nurse calls my name and escorts me to an exam room. This time, I settle into an upholstered chair rather than on the examining table.

Calming Gynecologist walks in and takes a seat next to me, an empathetic look on his face. He's about the same age as Doctor Doofus, but with a distinguished—rather than odd-ball—appearance.

"I'm sorry to hear you have breast cancer."

I immediately burst into sobs, grateful he seems willing to help. "The… radiologist…said…" I stop for a minute, trying to gain control over my disjointed speech.

Calming Gynecologist passes me a box of tissues. I feel as thankful as if he'd handed me a strand of pearls.

"He…said…that…I…I…I…should…get…a…breast…MRI." The gulps between each word grow even more pronounced.

"But…my…primary…care…doctor…said…it's…not…standard…protocol!"

"It's okay," he says. "I can order one for you."

"Thank you!" I blow my nose, making an unladylike honk. "But I don't understand. My PCP went to an Ivy League Medical School! Everyone says he's brilliant."

"Most of the time you don't want one of those guys," he says. "Their egos get in the way."

He glances at my chart, then meets my eyes. "What can I do to help you today? You must have lots of questions."

"Dozens." I'm comforted that his kind expression doesn't change, even though it's evident I may take up a big chunk of his time.

I start to ask my most pressing questions, such as which breast surgeon to see and where I should go to be treated. He gives me names of breast surgeons, oncologists, plastic surgeons, and internists he recommends.

"Should I go to a large cancer center downtown or one of the National Comprehensive Cancer Institutes? I don't think I want to be operated on by a general surgeon or at a community hospital. I want an oncology surgeon."

"Hmm," Calming Gynecologist replies. "I don't know any physicians at the NCCIs. But the doctors I mentioned are excellent and highly-regarded. I think you'd be in good hands at one of the major cancer centers downtown."

I go through my list of remaining questions. "Do you think I'll need chemotherapy?"

"That's a question you'll have to ask your oncologist. But I wouldn't be surprised if it's recommended. You're still pretty young for this." He shakes his head in dismay. "You know, a couple of weeks ago I had another patient in her mid-40s. Her routine mammogram picked up cancer too. Seems like it's happening at younger ages these days."

I nod in agreement and wonder why that is. *Is it because we are living more carcinogenic lives? Or because tumors are being detected earlier due to more sensitive screening technology?*

My breathing has returned to normal. I'm feeling less distraught.

"Anything else I can do for you today?" he asks when I finally flip my notebook to a blank page.

"The breast MRI?"

"No problem." He pulls out a form from a desk drawer. "I'll write the order right now."

I thank him profusely, and he tells me to call if I have any more questions. He also hands me a prescription for valium—for which I didn't ask—but that he apparently thinks I could use.

Divine Secret: Find physicians who are both smart and nice!

It's your body, so you have every right to ask questions and get answers. Don't let a doctor brush off your concerns or act condescending. It's perfectly fine to "fire" a physician who's not the right fit. You must be your own best advocate.

7

A Spoonful of Sugar Helps the Medicine Go Down

Feeling a great deal calmer, I drop off my prescription at the drugstore. Maybe I *could* use some Valium, my emotions still raw and precarious. I drive to a friend's house to pick up Larissa and ring the doorbell.

As she greets me, Kathleen's smile evaporates. "Joanna, are you okay?"

I've stopped crying, but my bloodshot eyes and mottled complexion must have tipped her off. Kathleen is super-intelligent and wired with innate wisdom, so I sometimes find myself confiding in her.

"Not really. I have breast cancer."

"Oh, no!" She motions me to come inside. "I'm so sorry."

"I just found out Friday. There's a lot I don't know yet."

"What can I do?"

"Watching Larissa is a big help."

"Anytime." She shakes her head. "I can't believe this. Did you find a lump?"

"No. Something didn't look right on my mammogram."

When Larissa ambles over with her My Little Pony backpack, we stop talking. She's so little, still in preschool. I don't want her to overhear anything.

I stop at the pharmacy on my way home. I give Ryan an update on my appointments, then we go through the motions of making dinner and washing dishes, trying to pretend every-thing is normal.

After Larissa's in bed, I pop a Valium and lock myself in the bathroom. Burying my face in a soft towel, I run water in the tub to cover the sound of my crying.

I feel drained already and it's just the beginning! How am I going to get through this?

As the pill kicks in, I start to feel a tiny bit braver. Usually, I'm a whistling-in-the-dark kind of girl and don't want to admit when I'm terrified. I remember walking home from elementary school with a classmate when boys started throwing dirt clods at us. My friend cried, but I took my Mary Poppins umbrella and whacked one boy upside the head. From then on, the mean kids left us alone.

And I take after Mom, who doesn't like to show fear. Once, on an executive Outward Bound–style rafting trip, she and a male colleague were tossed overboard and almost drowned. Rescued from the whitewater torrent, Mom kept it together but noticed her coworker struggling to control his emotions.

"Oh, damn it!" she yelled, holding up her hand to divert attention.

Everyone turned to her in alarm.

"I broke a nail!"

Even when I'm really scared and just bluffing, I vow to grip humor like a baseball bat and take a swing at cancer whenever I can.

～

The next morning, I see my friends Liz and Hannah at pre-school drop-off.

"Did your biopsy go okay?" Liz asks.

Liz and I joke sometimes about living parallel lives. We have the same quirky sense of humor and are both married to engi-neer-types who don't always share our liberal arts perspective.

"Not really," I answer. "I have breast cancer."

They are stunned into silence, their expressions ashen.

"Thanks for asking." Apparently, my Southern-fried manners are on autopilot.

"You know we're here for you," Liz says. "Every step of the way."

"Wow, I didn't expect to hear this. Let us help however we can," adds Hannah. "Will works with lots of surgeons."

"Oh, yeah." I remember that as a nurse anesthetist, Hannah's husband Will would have some good recommendations. "I'll definitely be asking his advice. I don't know much at this point."

"Of course we'll help with childcare and meals," Liz adds. "But I think we should focus on keeping your spirits up. Take you to coffee or lunch before every procedure or treatment."

"That sounds great." Lots of people can bring over lasagna, but not everyone can make me laugh like they do.

～

At this point, I've told Ryan, Mom, Kathleen, Hannah, and Liz that I have breast cancer. I'm hesitant to share the news with too many people, because doing so makes it all too real. I'm not ready for the sneaking glances at my bust line. I don't want to be an object of pity. And I don't want to answer questions.

Ryan and I are supposed to leave for our kid-free trip to Hilton Head, but I wonder whether we should go.

"Will we even enjoy it? I can't forget about the cancer."

"I know that." Ryan takes my hand. "The months ahead are going to be rough. The trip will give us time to think. And to talk without the kids around."

"Maybe you're right."

"Think of it as a little calm before the storm."

～

Before I finish packing, I go to the bookstore to buy some good reference books. I thought I had a baseline understanding of cancer, but there's so much more for me to learn. It's one heck

of a medical alphabet soup:
Invasive cancer or in-situ cancer?
Ductal, lobular or inflammatory?
Hormone-positive or hormone-negative?
Localized or metastatic?
Her2/positive, Her2/negative or triple negative?
Yikes, how am I ever going to understand all of this?
Ever since I was a child, I thought I could find an answer
to any problem in a book. Whatever obstacles I faced—failed
romances, broken friendships, parenting challenges—I always
trusted that the right reference guide would solve everything.
But this time it seems like the more I learn, the more questions
I have.

~

Finally, we load suitcases and drop the kids at my parents'
house. On the drive to Hilton Head, I'm constantly on my cell,
gathering information. Midway, we stop for gas and a soda.
    While Ryan is filling up our vehicle, I browse through the
periodicals rack. Tucked between body-building and sports car
magazines is *Beyond,* a glossy publication about breast cancer
with Brett Favre's wife, a survivor, on the cover.
    Is this some weird sign from above?
    I buy a copy and show it to Ryan. "Look what I found! A mag-
azine about breast cancer at a truckstop!"
    "Really?" He glances at the cover. "That's strange."
    I start to flip through the magazine, curious about what I'll
find.
    "Honey, I know your instinct is to research everything," he
says. "But I hope you'll take a mental break."
    "Okay." I sigh, slipping *Beyond* to the bottom of my stack of
beach reading material. I figure I can hide it inside a *Vanity Fair*
and he'll never know the difference.

~

We finally arrive at our destination. Thanks to Ryan's hotel points program, we get a few freebie nights at an upscale high-rise, much swankier than the sprawling, family-friendly resort we stay at with the kids. A porter piles our luggage on a baggage rack, along with grocery bags of drinks and snacks we've brought to avoid exorbitant mini-bar and room service prices. While Ryan gets our room key, I check my e-mail.

There's a message from a couple at our church. The husband is a family physician and the wife's a nurse, so I'd e-mailed them asking about surgeons and specialists. They've sent me a list of names and assurance I'll be in their prayers.

I'll take all the prayers I can get. I believe in God, but I'm usually too hard-headed to ask Him for help. Plus, when I reach the Pearly Gates, I'll have an even longer list of questions than I had for Doctor Doofus. I grew up in the Bible-Belt, where people will pray for something as mundane as a good parking spot. I guess with all of the terrible situations in the world—genocide, starvation, earthquakes—I feel awkward bothering the Big Guy with my piddling problems. I know He's the Great Multi-Tasker, but it always seems like other people need His attention more than I do.

But now that I have a cancer diagnosis, I don't mind bugging Him.

Divine Secret: Learn all you can about the enemy.

Don't be daunted by the unfamiliar terms. Learn medical terminology related to cancer so that you can better understand your pathology report and treatment options. Get physician recommendations from your nurse navigator or Pink Sisters who've faced the same battle.

Some reference books:

♦ *Living Through Breast Cancer,* by Carolyn Kaelin, M.D., M.P.H. with Francesca Coltrera

- *Navigating Breast Cancer: A Guide for the Newly Diagnosed*, by Lillie D. Shockney, R.N., B.S., M.A.S., Administrative Director, Johns Hopkins Breast Center
- *Dr. Susan Love's Breast Book*, by Susan M. Love, M.D. and Karen Lindsey

Life's a Beach

July 2007

H ere I sit poolside, surrounded by women in bikinis, tankinis, and skirted maillots. *Have any of them had breast cancer?* After all, no one has a pink ribbon glued to her forehead.

Partially hidden behind my magazine and sunglasses, I discreetly check out bust lines. Most of the teenage girls have fabulous figures, but probably fret that they are not a size 0. In a few decades, they'll realize that cellulite was *so* not a problem at age 17.

A rotund, dark-haired woman with a thick Russian accent sprawls on a nearby lounge chair. Playing chess with her husband, she stretches forward to move a rook, her v-neck suit revealing abundant milky-white, pillow-like cleavage.

A slender, tanned middle-aged woman in a white bikini and bejeweled sandals walks by. She has golden highlights in her hair, a French manicure and pedicure, plus a pair of unnaturally perky breasts which seem to defy gravity. *Silicone, perhaps?*

I scan the crowd, wondering: Can you tell when someone is wearing a prosthetic? After surgery, would scars show in a swimsuit? Are survivors limited to certain modest, high-necked styles?

Thinking about limitations in bathing suit fashion is trivial, but easier than thinking about my uncertain future. Everyone dies sooner or later, but I'd definitely prefer later. *My kids need me!* I'm not a perfect mom, but nobody could love them more.

Alex, our first-born, is starting high school. I remember his first word, first step, first loose tooth. The time he made a volcano for the science fair, caught a game-winning pop fly, went off to Space Camp. He has so many milestones ahead: learning to drive, attending the prom, graduating from high school. *What if I'm not around to witness them?*

Nick is starting middle school, that precarious stage between childhood and adolescence. I can vividly recall how he taught himself to ride a bike, surprising us with his skill, and when he painted a bouquet of flowers on canvas for me one Mother's Day. He's fearless and extroverted, so I worry the next few years will be turbulent, until his moral compass sends him in the right direction. *What if I'm not around to love and encourage him?*

Larissa, only five, is starting kindergarten. She was ten months old on adoption day, so we've only had four years together. It's heartbreaking to think that she could lose her mother for a second time. *If I died, how well would she remember me?*

I love my kids so much; I wish I could always spare them pain.

Ryan pulls his watch out of our tote bag. "Hey, where do you want to go for dinner?"

His question snaps me out of my ruminations, so we discuss several options: a Caribbean-themed seafood restaurant or a Mexican place overlooking a marina. I want to push the gloom away and have a fun, romantic time, but I can't shake the dark clouds.

We return our beach towels and head inside to shower. I change into black capris, strappy sandals, and a new blouse. Ryan sets the camera timer and places it on the dresser. He sits beside me on the couch and we hold our pose as the flash goes off. Will our smiles look fixed and fake, our eyes reflecting sadness and anxiety?

We choose the trendy seafood place. Waiting for our table, we sip wine in the bar. Trying not to talk about the evil, ugly elephant in the room, it's difficult to keep the conversation going. I know Ryan's having a hard time. He's attempting that mental compartmentalizing thing guys do. But I can't stop thinking about the hulking pink monster.

The wait-list buzzer beeps, breaking our awkward silence.

Once seated, Ryan holds up his wine glass. "To us."

We clink glasses and compare how different it is to vacation sans children.

"We don't have to watch cartoons," I say.

"Or go to restaurants with free crayons."

"Or lug toys to the beach."

"Let's try to have a good time while we're here." Ryan reaches for my hand.

"Agreed." I force myself to smile. When the waitress brings our menus, I order a second glass of wine, which I seldom do.

"Everything will be okay," he says, a faraway look in his eyes. "It has to be."

$\sim$

The next morning, Ryan and I ride bikes on the island's winding paths. We stop where alligators and turtles usually congregate, sunning on the grassy banks. Today, all we see is a trio of turtles.

We pedal past the pond, a golf course, residential streets, farther than we've ever gone before. I wonder what it would be like to live here fulltime. Would we start to take the power and majesty of the ocean for granted?

I think of the movie *Beaches*, where the Barbara Hershey character spends her last days at the Jersey shore, wrapped up in blankets on a chaise lounge. She tells her former BFF, played by Bette Midler, that she's dying and asks her friend to raise her daughter. Talk about a blatant tear-jerker!

Feeling uncomfortable emotions bubbling to the surface, I force myself to turn my thoughts from depressing movies of the past to the gorgeous scenery of today. Physically, it feels good to be in the warm sun, shaded at times by the leafy foliage, caressed by the cool ocean breeze. As I pedal, I feel strong, healthy, and resolute.

How can I feel so good yet have a deadly disease?

As we ride around the island, I vow to do whatever it takes to kick some cancer butt. Maybe it's not a cinematic moment, like Scarlett O'Hara digging for potatoes with her bare hands, shaking her fist at the sky, but while I steer around pedestrians and palm trees—as God is my witness—I vow to take the treatment path giving me the best odds of meeting my great-grandchildren.

～

We return the bikes, the sun now high in the sky. Back in our room to change into swimsuits, I check my e-mail and voice-mail. Will, Hannah's husband, has sent me a list of breast surgeons. Many of the names are familiar, also recommended by my other sources.

What do I do? Who should I call first?

I'm struggling over where to go for treatment, confused by a few well-meaning but conflicting opinions.

My first inclination has been to contact one of the large, prestigious National Comprehensive Cancer Institutes (NCCI) in the Mid-Atlantic or Southeast region. I'd receive top-notch care, but getting back and forth for frequent appointments, surgeries, and treatments would be a logistical headache. Plus, I've been warned—by someone trying to be helpful—not to go to *any* teaching hospital in July, the month medical facilities welcome their brand-spanking new residents. I agree; I don't really want some pimply medical student standing over me with a shaky knife.

Still, why would someone tell me NOT to go to a world-renowned cancer center? This doesn't make sense. Or does it?

We live in a suburb adjacent to a fairly large city, so the oncology surgeons downtown are probably quite good. Maybe that would make more sense. I have recommendations from people I trust. I scan the list and pick up the phone.

"Why don't you go ahead to the pool?" I urge Ryan.

"Nah, I'll wait for you." He settles in a chair, skimming a copy of *USA Today*, while I dial the number. The first oncology surgeon on my list, highly-regarded and female, is affiliated with the cancer center at one of the city's large hospitals. I cross my fingers, hoping for a quick appointment.

"I'm sorry," the receptionist explains. "The doctor is not accepting any new patients at this time."

"Oh," I answer, feeling deflated that Dr. Popular is not an option. "Thanks, anyway."

My heart sinks as I put down the phone. *How can an oncology surgeon turn a cancer patient away?*

Ryan looks at me, a question written on his face.

"No luck," I tell him.

I dial again, this time to reach a male oncology surgeon whom Will and Calming Gynecologist have both recommended. His receptionist tells me the first available appointment for Rock Star Surgeon is almost six weeks away.

What do I do? Should I look for a doctor who could operate sooner?

I look at Ryan and shake my head. I feel sick to my stomach.

I can't wait that long! Every day is a day the cancer keeps growing!

But on the other hand, I want someone with oncology expertise, so I accept the appointment—expressing my anxiety about the long wait.

The receptionist transfers me to voicemail for the surgeon's nurse. I leave a message that I've heard such great things about their practice but really, really hope they can work me in earlier.

Hanging up, I wonder if I'm being a snob. Friendly Oncologist said a general surgeon could probably operate within a week. As a cancer patient at a community hospital, maybe I'd get bumped ahead of people wanting elective surgery. Or perhaps those operating rooms aren't so tightly scheduled.

By going with a breast oncology specialist—like Rock Star Surgeon—I'll have to wait in line with all of the other cancer patients, every one of us scared and worried, pinning our hopes on the doctor's expertise.

"What did they say?" Ryan asks.

"I have an appointment, but it's over a month away."

"That's a long time."

"Yeah," I sigh.

I notice a missed call icon from Friendly Oncologist, apparently replying to a recent e-mail I sent him. I return the call, halfway expecting it to go to voicemail, when he picks up.

As I say "Hello," Ryan folds up the newspaper and leans forward, listening to my side of the conversation. I recap my disastrous appointment with Doctor Doofus, the condescending PCP, and my confusion over what to do next.

"I'm sorry," he says. "Why don't you consider me your personal guide while everything gets figured out? I'm glad to share my opinions and can help you schedule referral appointments."

He's offering to keep the treatment ball in motion, passing it strategically, like he's my very own Steve Nash pounding the basketball court. *How lucky am I?* Friendly Oncologist has earned a brand new, more descriptive moniker—Dr. Point Guard!

"Is it okay to wait over a month just for an appointment?" I ask. "Or would it be smarter to find someone else and have the surgery as soon as possible?"

"That does seem like a long time," he says. "I can understand your concern, but I don't think a few weeks either way should make any appreciable difference in your outcome."

Dr. Point Guard validates my thoughts that, yes, once a malignancy has been found, you want it removed in a timely manner. He explains that tumors grow at different rates. Some are aggressive and spread rapidly, but many grow for years before they are large enough to be detected.

"At this point, based on the mammogram and biopsy results, your cancer is suspected to be pretty small, probably Stage I, perhaps less than one centimeter in size. If you prefer an oncology surgeon—rather than a general surgeon—I think you'll be okay to wait for an appointment."

Dr. Point Guard again offers to help me however possible while I decide on doctors and treatment paths.

I'm very grateful for his kindness.

I hang up and consider calling a surgeon at my community hospital for an earlier appointment. How can I wait a month, knowing that cancer is growing inside me, without losing my mind? Yet I really want a cancer specialist to operate.

As usual, I've googled myself into a frenzy, already thinking ahead to various scenarios if I end up having a mastectomy. From what I've read, many women are able to get "immediate" reconstruction, whereby a plastic surgeon works in tandem with the breast surgeon. However, reconstructive surgery is not your ordinary boob job. It takes a lot of time and specialized skills. Most regular plastic surgeons don't do them often.

Divine Secret: Be prepared to wait, and wait, and wait.

There's no quick and easy shortcut out of Cancerland; you might get stranded in Wait-and-Worryland. You'll have to wait for appointments, surgery dates, healing before treatment, lab test results, etc. Take a number and get used to it, girlfriend.

I might find a great general surgeon at the community hospital, but it's unlikely I'll find a local plastic surgeon specializing in reconstruction. Granted, choosing a cosmetic procedure is far less important than getting rid of the cancer, yet it's another consideration to factor in the decision-making process.

Since Ryan only heard my side of the conversation, I fill him in and lament my ever-increasing frustration.

"Screw it," I say. "Let's go to the pool. I could use a few of those tropical umbrella drinks."

I grab the sunscreen and a celebrity magazine, eager to worry about Brad, Angelina, and Jennifer rather than myself.

Meet and Greet with Rock Star Surgeon

W e try to salvage some fun and relaxation at the beach, but I keep running back to the room to use the phone and laptop. Then, I get a call from Rock Star Surgeon's office. There's been a cancellation, so they can work me in next week! *My groveling voicemail message worked!*

The last night, we go to the Mexican restaurant overlooking the marina. It's normally fun and upbeat to sit on the patio sipping margaritas, listening to Jimmy Buffett songs, and watching the boats dock. But our mood tonight is quiet and reflective.

After dinner, we browse in the island's biggest bookstore. I select a few novels and purchase a book of personal essays written by a group of breast cancer survivors. I read in the preface that the editor died before the book was complete, so her Pink Sisters finished it. *Stupid dumb-ass disease!*

∼

Driving home the next morning, Ryan wonders aloud what we should say to the kids. "When do you think we should tell them?"

"I don't know." I press my fingers against my temples, trying to ward off a brewing migraine. "Soon, I guess."

I don't want them to be scared. I want to promise that every-thing will be okay. *But will it?*

"We'd better not wait too long."

"Yeah, Nick's already asked why I've had so many doctor appointments."

We decide to keep quiet for a few more days, until after I see Rock Star Surgeon and have a better idea of my treatment plan.

$\sim$

Back home from the beach, I count down the days until my appointment with the oncology surgeon. Whenever the kids are at summer day camp or playing with friends, I peruse websites sponsored by the *American Cancer Society* and other reputable organizations, trying to make sense out of all these scientific, unfamiliar terms.

I'm thankful for the educational resources available today. Only decades ago, it was unthinkable to discuss cancer in polite company. Long before J.K. Rowling imagined Lord Voldemort, "cancer" was the original word one dared not speak.

Researching stuff is my natural tendency, so I begin to under-stand how cancers are categorized according to both stage and grade. Stages range from Stage 0 (non-invasive) to Stage IV (metastatic). Within these stages, there are sub-stages that delineate differences. In general, with Stage 0, often referred to as DCIS (Ductal Carcinoma In Situ), the cancer is contained within the breast ducts and has not yet gained the ability to spread to other parts of the body. *This is good!*

However, any other stage means you have invasive cancer. The size of the tumor and whether or not there is lymph node involvement determines whether you are Stage I, Stage II, or Stage III.

Stage IV means that the cancer has invaded other organs, most commonly bones, liver, or lungs. There is no Stage V. *This is not good.*

I'm hopeful my condition is early-stage, but there's no way to know for sure until after surgery and lab reports.

In addition to being staged, the cancer cells are assigned a grade by the pathologist. *I'd give mine an "F-minus" and after-school detention!* The grade helps predict the cancer's behavior, whether it can grow at an aggressive pace or if it's more indolent.

I learn that knowing whether your cancer is fueled by estrogen or progesterone is critical. Estrogen-responsive (ER+) or progesterone-responsive (PR+) cancer means that the tumor feeds off hormones, so taking birth control pills or hormone replacement therapy can be like pouring gasoline on a fire. Physicians usually advise women with ER+ and PR+ cancer to take tamoxifen if they are premenopausal, or another class of drugs, aromatase inhibitors (often called AIs), if they are postmenopausal. These drugs work by blocking estrogen or shutting down its production.

I read that while breast cancer is much less common in younger women, it tends to be more deadly. Statistically, without a strong family history of cancer, breast cancer is unlikely in your 20s or 30s. Unfortunately, this means that sometimes physicians will delay biopsying a lump, incorrectly assuming it's a benign cyst.

Sometimes the cancer is caught at a later stage since screening mammograms aren't recommended until age 40. Other times the cancer is more aggressive because it's fed by hormones younger women are still producing in greater quantities.

At age 45 and premenopausal, I fall under the "younger patient" category. Normally, it would be a treat for my ego to be considered "young," but this is one time I'd really like an AARP membership card.

I click the computer mouse to read about different surgical options. I research the differences between mastectomies and lumpectomies. Pros and cons of each surgery, such as length of recovery time, change in appearance, and loss of sensation. *Ugh!*

I study the possible side effects of chemotherapy and radiation, such as hair loss, nausea, brain fog, exhaustion, and nerve damage. *Double ugh!*

I'm learning more than I ever wanted to know.

Then, spurred by some reckless instinct—like jumping out of an airplane with a garage-sale sky-diving parachute—I google survival rates calculated by cancer stage and grade.

It takes me a moment to grasp the information.

Hmm.

The statistics look very good for early-stage, low-grade cancer patients, with about a 98% survival rate, yet they decline by stage. *But why are all the statistics based on a five-year term? Five years is nothing!* I want to dance at my daughter's wedding and argue with her about the catering menu. I want to spend time with my future grandchildren (at least until they need diaper changes or have grocery-store meltdowns).

Where are the reassuring survival rates for 20, 30, 40+ years of a cancer-free future?

I'm being sucked into a grim vortex of fear. My head spinning and stomach churning, I flounder for a distraction. *Got to find something else to think about, and quick—something less grim than survival statistics.*

Foobs. I'll research "foobs," the nickname some survivors give their fake boobs. *(Here's a shout-out to my brave Ta-Ta Sisters who've shared reconstruction photos!)* I have to be discreet, though. It would be awkward if the boys caught me looking at topless photos on the Internet.

I learn that the most common type of reconstruction is done with breast implants. *Not too certain this is for me.* I'm a little squeamish about silicone, not wanting to end up with some freakish Pamela Anderson–style pneumatic melons.

Then I read about a different type of procedure, where surgeons remove extra skin and fat from your abdomen to fashion a "foob." *What a great idea!* I've always had an ample belly, even in my teenaged years when I was still a single-digit size.

My eyes light up at the discovery of this option. I don't just have a muffin top, I've got the whole damn bakery going on! Surely there's plenty of potential foob material with which to work. Maybe a free tummy tuck will be my consolation prize for all of this cancer crap!

I start to daydream about how this might work. Okay, so life hands me lemons. But I won't just make lemonade, I'll make a fricking lemon-drop martini! By golly, when this is all over, I'll have a brand-spanking new set of foobs not yet undone by gravity and, for once in my life, a flat stomach.

Maybe my Extreme Cancer Makeover won't be so bad after all.

Next summer, I could ditch my matronly black maillot with the built-in support bra and the tummy-control panels for a cute little tankini. I'll stop hiding Twix bars in the cupboards like an alcoholic stashing vodka bottles in the toilet tank. I'll start running for exercise, not just to chase the ice-cream truck.

Who knows, maybe my plastic surgeon will be an absolute genius—the Beethoven of boob jobs, the Tchaikovsky of tummy tucks. I close my eyes and picture my new, slender self in a white string bikini, jogging along the surf on a tropical island as the cute surfer dudes stare in awe.

Yeah, right, like this is going to happen. I haven't worn a bikini since the 1970s, but a girl can always dream.

~

Ryan and I wait in the downtown oncology center for my appointment with Rock Star Surgeon. I keep re-reading my list of questions and clicking my pen. It's unnerving to be in a doctor's office that deals strictly with cancer patients. Some people are wearing bandannas or hats. A few are in wheelchairs, looking frail. Others appear perfectly healthy.

A petite brunette nurse, holding a clipboard, opens the door and calls my name.

"How are you feeling today?" she asks, as we walk down the corridor.

"Nervous, but eager to hear what the doctor says."

"I know it's scary," she says, patting my shoulder. "But I'm sure you'll feel much better after your appointment. The doctor always spends a lot of time with patients at their first consultation."

Caring Nurse escorts us into an exam room where Rock Star Surgeon makes his entrance. He's an attractive man with a pleasant demeanor, probably somewhere in his early to mid-40s.

"Good to meet you," he says, shaking my hand, then Ryan's.

"I've heard wonderful things about you!" I gush.

"Thanks, but don't believe everything you hear." With a self-deprecating smile, he directs us to sit at a small table with a flip chart. Pictured is a sketch of the female anatomy, labeling parts of the breasts and lymph nodes. He starts talking about the basics of breast cancer, which by this time I've researched extensively.

"It appears that your tumor is here, in the nine o'clock position," he says, pointing to an illustration. "You're a perfect candidate for lumpectomy, followed up by radiation."

I frown. I've read about lumpectomies, the removal of only the diseased area instead of the entire breast. But I'm not totally convinced that it's right for me. "How can you be sure of getting all the cancer out?"

"Clear margins. Which means the pathologist looks at the borders of the tissue extracted," he explains. "If there are any abnormal cells within one centimeter of the edge, I'll go back in for a re-excision to take out more tissue. This finding is not uncommon. It happens for about fifteen percent of patients. On rare occasions, I'll do a third excision."

A second or third operation?

"Many times you'll get a very good cosmetic result from lumpectomy, with little change to the breast except a small scar," he explains. "The appearance will vary depending on the size and location of the tumor. A lumpectomy from the lower half of the breast or near the nipple generally causes more disfigurement. I think in your case, you'd get a good result."

Rock Star Surgeon then tells us that patients choosing lumpectomy follow up with a series of radiation treatments.

"I don't know. With a mastectomy, I wouldn't worry as much about the cancer coming back."

"Let me explain. All the studies have shown there is no difference in outcome—meaning survival—when a woman has a choice between lumpectomy plus radiation or mastectomy."

"That's encouraging," adds Ryan.

"The patient choosing lumpectomy does have a *slightly* higher risk of having a *local recurrence*—meaning cancer returning to the breast near the original site—because there's more breast tissue remaining."

"This wouldn't change my survival rate?"

"No," he explains. "Because with survival, we're talking about whether or not the cancer has spread to your other organs. The chances of *distant recurrence*—meaning metastatic cancer—is the same whether the patient chooses lumpectomy plus radiation or mastectomy."

"Hmm." I get that he's trying to explain that a reappearance of cancer cells still isolated in my breast would not kill me, like they could if they spread to my lungs or liver. *But who wants to face breast cancer a second time? What are the odds of this happening?*

"Even with mastectomy," Rock Star Surgeon continues, "there's still a small amount of breast tissue left behind. Chances are slim, but cancer could recur locally even in that situation."

It's starting to sink in that I'll always have a risk of recurrence—either as a local or metastatic event. With my anxious nature, it's going to be hard to keep this bogeyman in the closet.

Rock Star Surgeon directs our attention to another illustration to explain the sentinel node procedure.

"Before surgery, a radiologist will inject your nipple area with an iodine dye to indicate the drainage path of the lymph nodes."

Ouch!

"Therefore," he points to the flip chart, "only a few nodes—the sentinels—need to be excised unless we find cancer cells in them. In the past, lymph node dissection often caused lymph-edema, which is chronic pain and swelling in the arm. Sentinel node biopsy has greatly reduced this risk."

I nod to show him I'm listening carefully.

"If the cancer has spread to your lymph nodes, you'll need another operation, called an axillary dissection, to remove more nodes. We won't know for sure until we get the complete pathology report, but the sentinel node status is a very good indicator."

Rock Star Surgeon starts talking about following lumpectomy with radiation therapy, explaining the benefits and potential side effects.

"The sentinel node thing sounds good," I interject. "But I'm not keen on radiation."

A fleeting look of irritation crosses his face. I can tell he's a little put off by my interrupting his presentation. But I can't help it! He's talking extensively, almost exclusively, about lumpectomy, getting clear margins, radiation.

"I'm not sure about the lumpectomy. I think I want a mastectomy. A bilateral, actually. With DIEP or TRAM, one of those immediate breast reconstruction procedures that'll give me the bonus tummy tuck."

He seems a bit stunned, as if I've just placed my order for a double bacon cheeseburger with curly fries.

"I want to reduce the chances of cancer coming back," I say. "I don't want to worry about another tumor showing up in my breast. In either one. Besides," I joke, gesturing toward my chest, "these gals are past their prime. Already reached their expiration date."

"Well," he says, looking at me as if I'm a bit of a nutcase, unsure whether he's supposed to laugh. "A mastectomy isn't really necessary. You're a perfect candidate for lumpectomy."

Across the table I catch Ryan's sharp glance reminding me to be a good girl and listen to the renowned doctor. I sigh and tell myself to keep an open mind.

"Lumpectomy is the gold standard for treatment today," Rock

Star Surgeon reassures us. "If you're a good candidate, as in your case, then there's no difference in survival rates."

I listen as he reiterates the positive aspects of lumpectomy again. Outpatient procedure. No overnight hospital stay. Less disfigurement. Less loss of sensation. A quicker and easier recovery than mastectomy.

Hmm. Breast-conserving surgery and a shorter recovery would make it easier to keep my cancer under the radar. Fewer people would have to know. I could even have a lumpectomy scheduled as soon as next week, then get the doctor's approval to go on a long-planned cruise with Ryan's family two weeks later. I admit this option sounds good.

Ryan is nodding, encouraging me to listen to Rock Star Surgeon.

Sigh. I want to choose my treatment plan based on knowledge, not fear. I sought out a highly-regarded doctor, so I should probably take his advice.

"Think it over," the doctor says. "In the meantime, talk with my surgery scheduler. She can also set up an appointment with a plastic surgeon if you decide on a mastectomy."

Divine Secret: It can be really hard making treatment decisions.

Nobody warns you how tough it can be to make treatment decisions. Sometimes your gut instincts contradict what your brain is telling you. Don't be afraid to seek out second or even third opinions. Brilliant doctors don't always offer the same advice or opinion.

Rock Star Surgeon bids us goodbye. He's spent an hour talking with us, which I greatly appreciate.

The efficient and pretty surgery scheduler comes in the room to set up a tentative date and time for lumpectomy, telling us to let her know what we decide.

I leave the exam room with a thick folder of information and a vaguely uneasy feeling. Is this because I'm an overly-nervous, neurotic patient wanting to use a bazooka instead of a flyswatter to kill a gnat? Or is it gut instinct to which I should listen?

Or maybe I'm just disappointed that I might be missing out on the free tummy tuck.

Sending Out an S.O.S.

Uncertain and confused, I attend a support group at the local community hospital. Despite scheduling a lumpectomy, I feel uneasy and can't figure out why. Maybe some advice from women who've *been there, done that* would help.

Wearing a long skirt with a crunchy-granola vibe and ergonomic sandals, Faux-Hippie Facilitator asks each attendee to introduce herself. Several dominate the conversation, including Slender Fashionista, an attractive, stylish lady in her 60s. Wearing a green cardigan set, preppy capris, and cute sandals that show off her pedicure, she shares her reluctance to take a medication her oncologist has prescribed.

Cat Fanatic, a heavy-set older woman in a fuzzy kitten t-shirt and stretch pants, has an arm as swollen as an elephant's trunk. *Yikes!* I've read about how lymphedema—painful swelling— may occur after removal of the lymph nodes, but I never imagined anything this bad! She's also discouraged about other health problems that require her to use a walker and an oxygen tank. I feel guilty for fixating on her enlarged arm rather than her warm hazel eyes.

Glancing around the circle of twelve chairs, no one seems close to my age, with the exception of Sensible Survivor, who appears to be in her late 40s or early 50s, dressed in a camp-style shirt, khaki slacks, and Easy Spirit shoes, with thick plastic glasses and a no-nonsense hair style.

"Who would like to share a concern?" asks Faux-Hippie Facilitator.

"My doctor keeps telling me to take this medication," complains Slender Fashionista. "But I don't want to."

"Why not?" Cat Fanatic says.

"Can you tell us what you're feeling?" asks Faux-Hippie Facilitator.

"I've never been on a daily medication before," she says. "Taking it is just one more reminder of the cancer."

"The medication you're talking about is an aromatase inhibitor, prescribed to prevent recurrence, right?" asks Sensible Survivor.

"Yes," admits Slender Fashionista.

"Are you comfortable talking to your oncologist about this?" asks Faux-Hippie Facilitator.

"I've *talked* to him several times. He's not happy with me."

"Maybe you should listen to him," responds Cat Fanatic. "You don't want the cancer coming back."

"I don't know," replies Slender Fashionista. "I'm scared of the side effects. I've heard others say it causes joint pain and weight gain."

"Maybe that won't happen," suggests Sensible Survivor.

Slender Fashionista shakes her head. "I don't know."

The conversation stays on this topic for endless minutes. I know I'm supposed to be all empathetic and supportive, but the clock is ticking. I need some answers!

"Maybe you could try the medication for a few weeks?" I suggest. "You could stop if the side effects are too bad."

"Well, maybe so…"

"May I bring up a different subject?" I ask. "I'd really like to hear everyone's opinions."

"Go ahead," urges Cat Fanatic.

"I'm trying to decide between lumpectomy and mastectomy.

My surgeon is recommending lumpectomy, but my gut instinct keeps resisting. What did you do?"

I conduct an informal poll around the circle. Only two chose lumpectomies. This surprises me. The rest had either a single or double mastectomy. A few had lumpectomies initially, without clear margins, before deciding to remove the entire breast.

Frankly, the idea of multiple surgeries for the same tumor sounds terrible. I imagine myself waking up in the recovery room every day, as if I'm Bill Murray in some grim pink-ribbon re-make of *Groundhog Day*.

Two of the women explain why they decided on mastectomy from the start. One cites a strong family history, and another says she didn't want the radiation treatments recommended after lumpectomy.

"What about reconstruction? I'm interested in one of those tissue-transfer techniques."

Most of the women shake their heads.

"I was so small-chested that I didn't bother," says Slender Fashionista.

"I didn't do reconstruction," adds Cat Fanatic. "And I can't find a decent prosthesis. They don't make them big enough."

She didn't have to tell us this, because the lack of symmetry underneath her kitty t-shirt is glaringly obvious. I've been trying all night to avert my eyes, but I can't stop stealing glances, as if she were an overturned car on a highway median. *How discouraging it must be when every casual observer can see the destruction cancer has wreaked upon your body.*

Divine Secret: Check out the array of breast forms and lymphedema products now available.

American Breast Care, Amoena Life, Anita Care, and Trulife offer breast forms to match women of virtually any shape or size. If, like Cat Fanatic, you're still struggling to find a good fit, investigate radiantimpressions.com for a custom prosthesis. Also, check out LympheDIVAs.com, a company that offers stylish, custom-fit compression sleeves and gauntlets to help prevent the painful swelling of lymphedema.

"I had reconstruction after chemo," says Sensible Survivor. "But I'm not happy. It was done with an implant and doesn't look anything like my other breast."

Gee, that's one of the issues I've been reading about.

Apparently, reconstruction with implants looks best on younger women who are modestly endowed. While a natural breast will age and succumb to gravity over the years, the one with the implant remains perky and upright. For better symmetry, you can get a breast lift and/or a reduction of the remaining natural breast, but results vary, depending on the surgeon's skill and the patient's anatomy.

As Faux-Hippie Facilitator ends the meeting, everyone encourages me to come back. Although I appreciate their friendliness and candor, I'm still frustrated. I'd been hoping to meet someone in my situation. A kindred spirit, a busy soccer-mom with young kids and a preference for shopping at Banana Republic for a few more years before graduating to Chico's.

∼

I continue to feel uncertain. Dr. Point Guard and Rock Star Surgeon keep telling me lumpectomy is the gold standard, yet the idea of possibly undergoing multiple excisions and radiation treatments unnerves me.

The next time Dr. Point Guard calls, I bring up the subject again.

"You're an excellent candidate for lumpectomy," he reiterates. "All the studies have shown survival rates are equivalent whether you do lumpectomy plus radiation or mastectomy. With the lumpectomy route, there is a higher risk of local recurrence, but your outcome—as in survival rate—is the same."

Blah, blah, blah. I've heard all this before. I understand that from a treatment perspective, lumpectomy seems a wise choice. *But the greater odds of a local recurrence bother me.*

"I know," I answer. "But I keep thinking about a bilateral, a complete teardown and reconstruction. The girls are showing their age, anyway."

Maybe this is sort of like deciding not to renovate an old house. Just bulldoze the site and build a sparkling new McMansion, a choice that may cause disagreement, but is a valid option nonetheless.

"Your other breast has no signs of cancer," he replies, exasperation creeping into his voice. "I don't advise the removal of a healthy organ."

A *healthy organ?* I guess I've never really thought of my breast as an "organ," *per se.* It's not like a liver or heart, something I absolutely need to survive. There's no National Breast Donor Registry. (But if there were, I can imagine thousands of women signing up, eager to donate their excess abdominal fat.)

This isn't the first time my breasts have let me down. As a new mother, despite coaching by lactation consultants and the La Leche League, every time I tried to breastfeed Alex, we'd both end up crying. When his weight plateaued—and the pain of cracked nipples got so bad I was cursing under my breath rather than whispering sweet endearments—I knew it was time for a bottle.

We end the call. I tell Dr. Point Guard I'll think about it some more, but I'm frustrated by our differing opinions. Amputating a hand or leg, now that would cause me some physical challenges. Taking off my breasts? *Not so much.*

I'm starting to wonder if part of this is a guy thing. Male doctors seem particularly appalled at the idea of removing a cancer-free breast unless there's strong incentive to do so, such as a confirmed BRCA mutation, a gene that means you have higher than average odds of developing breast cancer. Yet I've heard a number of women—including some female physicians—say that if they were diagnosed, they'd want both breasts removed *pronto.*

Is this a knee-jerk panicked reaction from the women? Or does it indicate men's excessive reverence for boobs? My brain is starting to hurt. *Why can't I get my head and heart to reach a consensus?*

~

Still confused and anxious, I return to Rock Star Surgeon's office. After my initial appointment, Caring Nurse had urged me to come back anytime I needed an empathetic listener and sounding board. She's blocked out time to help me sort through my concerns.

Upon my arrival, she escorts me to a private exam room. "What's going on? Tell me what you're thinking."

"I keep hearing I should get a lumpectomy, but I don't know."

Despite trying to hold it together, my eyes tear. Caring Nurse leans forward and hands me a tissue.

"It's okay to feel this way," she reassures me. "Many patients struggle with this decision."

"I'm trying so hard to figure it out."

"Anything in particular that might help you decide?"

"Can you tell me if I'm ER and PR positive or negative?"

She studies my file for a few minutes, shaking her head. "For some reason, the biopsy report doesn't say."

What? It's not in the report?

I burst into great gulping sobs. *Great! I haven't been operated on yet but already there's an oversight!* I can't help but think of all those crazy news stories I've heard about medical mishaps. Like a surgeon removing someone's left—not the right—I mean *correct*— body part. *Huh?* Or an in-vitro procedure with a stranger's sperm sample, not your husband's. Perhaps a surgical instrument left behind, only to show up in an X-ray decades later.

"Don't worry," she says, patting my shoulder. "I'll take care of it. It must have been overlooked. I'll call the pathology lab."

"I really need to know!"

"It should've been in the report, but I don't see how your hormone status would affect the decision whether or not to have a mastectomy."

I dab my eyes and take a deep breath. "I've read that if you have ER- or PR-negative cancer, your body doesn't respond to adjuvant treatment drugs like tamoxifen. If your tumor tests hormone negative, your only big-gun post-surgical ammunition is chemotherapy and radiation."

"Yes, in general terms, that's true."

"So, if I'm ER- or PR-negative, I'd almost definitely do chemo. Then I'd worry about a recurrence in the breast tissue left behind. What if there were a few stray cancer cells the radiation didn't get that could spread?"

"Okay, I understand where you're coming from. But let's think positively. First off, the majority of breast cancers—about seventy-five percent—are hormone-positive. If that's your case, then depending on the tumor size and node status, you may not need chemotherapy at all. Treatments are becoming more and more tailored to the individual patient."

I nod and sniffle.

"There's a new genetic test for hormone-positive patients called Oncotype. It predicts whether or not you're likely to benefit from chemo. After surgery, we'll send out a tissue sample and their lab will evaluate, based on unique tumor markers, your personal risk of recurrence. If your score is low, then you may forgo chemo."

I sigh and wad up my tissue, noncommittal to her positive-thinking approach. *Can I trust this test?* Chemo's no fun, but I'm afraid of what might happen if I skipped it.

How would I feel if the cancer ever came back?

"I'll follow up with the lab," Caring Nurse assures me. "I'll call you as soon as we get results. In the meantime, go talk to a plastic surgeon and try not to worry."

🔒 *DS*

Divine Secret: Medical professionals make mistakes, too.

Doctors, nurses, lab technicians, etc. are human; ergo, they make mistakes from time to time. Even at the best facilities, errors and oversights happen. Ask questions if something seems wrong. You have the right to request copies of all of your exam results and lab tests. Consider getting a second or even third opinion on pathology reports, treatment strategies, or surgery options.

Me? Not worry?

I drive home, drained and ticked off at the pathology lab. *How could they let my hormone-receptor test slip through the cracks?* It's one thing to make a mistake if you work in some random office and neglect to mail a package or forget to order a part for the assembly line. Maybe it causes financial loss or a factory shutdown. But still, it's not cancer. *People in the cancer business should not screw up!*

Dropping the Bombshell

Though I'm mentally exhausted from the turmoil, it's been only about two weeks since my diagnosis. We need to tell the kids, though we're both been dreading it. Next, I need to figure out who else to contact and how much to share.

Normally, I'm somewhat private. I share my concerns with close friends, but not the world at large. I know some women make extraordinary efforts to conceal their disease, buying a wig in their color and style to camouflage hair loss before it starts. Or they might take minimal sick days, tucking drainage bulbs in the waistband of their skirts, working before and after chemo or radiation treatments if possible. This approach keeps casual acquaintances from knowing your personal business. Maybe at one time I'd have considered this, but now I think some transparency is important for the sake of my children.

If Ryan and I are overly discreet, then the kids might think cancer is some sort of terrible secret. I want to protect them, but I can't completely alleviate their fears. I'm sure people will ask them how I'm doing. Maybe Alex and Nick will worry we aren't being completely honest. Word will get out anyway, since we're involved in a number of activities: school, sports, scouts, church, etc. I don't want the kids overhearing rumors.

When Larissa is playing at a friend's house, Ryan asks the boys to join us in the study. "Take a seat, guys." I look at them, working up my nerve. Taller than me, and fully a teenager, Alex has braces and a head of loose curls. As usual, Nick is wearing basketball shorts, his thick mop of hair underneath a baseball cap.

How will this experience change them?

"What's going on?" asks Alex.

Ryan and I exchange nervous glances.

"There's something we need to tell you." I stare at the wood grain of the desk, unwilling to make eye contact. "I've had a lot of doctor appointments lately."

"Yeah, why is that?" Nick asks.

I take a deep breath and look up. "I've been diagnosed with breast cancer."

The boys look stunned. Alex's mouth gapes open. Nick starts to snicker, shocked at the word "breast" spoken aloud, but stops himself and wrings his hands.

"The good news is we caught it early."

I glance at Ryan. He's silent, struggling to keep a calm and confident demeanor.

"Are you going to be okay?" Nick asks, his blue eyes clouded with worry.

"Yes, honey," I say, hoping this is a truthful answer. "I'll need surgery and maybe some radiation or chemotherapy treatments, but the doctors think I'll be fine."

"I can't believe this," mutters Alex, shaking his head.

"You guys need to know. But Larissa's too young to understand. We'll explain to her that Mommy needs surgery a few days before it happens."

"The next few months will be tough, but we'll get through them," Ryan adds.

"I have very good doctors," I reassure them, trying to erase the fear and doubt scrawled across their faces. I remind Nick that Dr. Point Guard is his former basketball coach. That he's a very smart man.

"We'll need you guys to help out more," Ryan says. "And Nana will be coming to stay while Mom is in the hospital."

"It's going to be okay." I choke down the lump in my throat.

We stand up, embracing the boys in big hugs. After they go upstairs to resume a video game and Ryan leaves the room, I slump down in the chair, emotionally spent and exhausted. The tears I've been fighting back finally win.

～

Every time I tell someone, the cancer becomes more real. Although we've only told our families and close friends, I'm already tired of talking about it. We still need to tell the kids' teachers and our friends back in Texas, where I grew up. I've got to figure out *how* to share the news. I hate seeing furrowed brows and sorrowful eyes. Everyone will want to be supportive, but I don't want to be the topic of every conversation. Also, I don't want Ryan barraged with questions, since this is sure to stir up bad memories.

How can I keep people updated and avoid answering the same questions over and over?

I know; I'll set up a blog.

I log onto *CaringBridge*, a free website for sharing information about personal health issues. Friends and family can read your updates and add encouraging remarks. They can check in and pass on good wishes without having to call.

Choosing a template of cheerful daisies for my *CaringBridge* page, I summarize my recent diagnosis. I add a few jokey comments—like how my breasts are now getting more attention than those belonging to a Hooters waitress—to lighten the gloomy message.

Hmm, who should I send the link to first?

For several reasons, our Adoption Travel Group comes to mind.

～

Though none of the families live nearby, we have a special bond. In February of 2003, we spent over two weeks in China welcoming our beautiful daughters. We met in Hong Kong and shared tiny postage-stamp sized photos of our daughters-to-be. Days later, we waited together in a hotel conference room in Nanchang, giddy with anticipation and happiness.

It was a magical moment that still takes my breath away, the instant when nine Chinese nannies marched into that conference room. Each held a baby girl dressed in multiple layers of clothes and wearing a laminated ID tag. It was an intimate and unforgettable experience, like being in a communal labor and delivery room. I held Larissa Jun Mei for the first time and knew she was mine forever.

We then spent two incredible weeks in Nanchang and Guangzhou, lingering over breakfast buffets, feeding our girls Cheerios and *congee*, a traditional Chinese rice porridge. We sat in the hallways of the hotel, playing with our daughters, delighting over their smiles as each girl grew to trust her "forever family."

Our travel group was diverse, including engineers, corporate executives, nurses, stay-at-home moms, teachers, an attorney, and even a casino pit dealer. All clients of the same adoption agency, we hailed from different areas of the country, but vowed to stay in touch. One dad even designed a pendant for each girl out of a golden medallion split into nine equal pieces, a physical reminder of our deep connection.

~

Less than a year after bringing our daughters home, I received a terrible message. One of the moms had a cancer recurrence. A beautiful and brainy attorney, Christine was a runner, a vegetarian, and in top physical condition. The last person you'd expect to face terminal illness.

After submitting adoption paperwork, but before receiving their long-awaited referral, Christine was diagnosed with a rare form of cancer (not breast cancer). However, by the time of the China adoption trip, she had completed treatment and they were optimistic about the future. So she and her husband decided to bring their daughter home to her big sister, grandparents, aunts, uncles, and cousins.

Not wanting to jeopardize the adoption, they kept things under wraps. While in China, Christine wore a cute blonde bob I never suspected was a wig. While she donned a scarf sometimes at the hotel, I never saw her in it and had no idea she was growing out post-chemo hair. Returning home, their family thought she'd beaten cancer. That is, until it spread to her bones, fracturing her femur.

～

Our travel group had been e-mailing back and forth for weeks, discussing dates and locations for a future reunion. Then I got a call from Christine.

"Hi, Joanna," she said. "Thanks for planning everything."

"I'm glad to," I replied. "How are you feeling these days?"

"I'm okay. Some days are better than others."

We talked about our daughters and how much they had grown. And about how we were looking forward to seeing the other families again.

"I wanted to talk to you about the reunion," she said. "Jeff and I would really like to have it this summer if possible. I don't know what things will be like next year. Or how easy it will be for me to travel then."

I concentrated on keeping my voice steady, lumbering through a fog of sadness. "No problem, Christine. We want to do what's best for your family."

～

In August 2004, seven of the nine families met in Myrtle Beach. Our daughters splashed in the pool and played in the sand. Christine, undergoing chemotherapy once again, donned a baseball cap to protect her scalp from the sun. Her spirit was strong; we all hoped she'd somehow beat this nasty disease.

In the ensuing months, every time Jeff sent an update, things were progressively worse. Despite lengthy hospitalizations and multiple surgeries, treatment was no longer effective, so Christine moved to hospice care. On Christmas Eve, her doctor let her go home from the hospital for 24 hours. What a bittersweet time it must have been, the joy of being home mixed with knowledge that it would be their last holiday together.

Christine passed away in February of 2005, less than two years after our adoption trip to China. She'd faced her disease with such courage and grace.

∼

Divine Secret: Plan your communications strategy.

Figure out who needs to know and how much to share. Would you welcome lots of phone calls or would you feel overwhelmed answering questions? Would you prefer to update people via e-mail or blog posts? There are several websites that offer free, easy-to-use web pages and blogs to people wanting to keep their friends and families updated on health situations:
- CaringBridge.org
- MyLifeline.org (cancer specific)
- CarePages.com

As parents of nine precious girls, we'd bonded with this group over both happiness and tragedy, so I knew they'd keep us lifted up in prayers and good wishes. Also, I have to confess that sharing the news with local friends and neighbors is a little too close to home. It's easier to start by telling the Adoption Group families; I won't run into them at the supermarket.

I type up an e-mail to our Adoption Travel Group, include a link to my *CaringBridge* page and hit "send."

My public battle against cancer officially begins.

Finding My Bosom Buddies

I need to find my tribe. Everyone I met at the local support group was nice, but I want to connect on a deeper level. I investigate several online communities, reading posts, asking a few tentative questions, when I find a place for me to belong in the *Young Survival Coalition*. Most members are under 40, so, at age 45, I'm a little long in the tooth, but I find them to be kindred spirits. Not yet an empty-nester or retiree, I share many of their concerns and perspectives.

Breast cancer is a lousy disease for anyone, but it can be a different animal when you're pre-menopausal. Although cancer in younger women is uncommon, it tends to be more aggressive. Sometimes told they're "too young" to have cancer, women in their 20s and 30s may not receive an accurate diagnosis until the disease has progressed to an advanced stage. Also, some subtypes of breast cancer are fueled by the hormones estrogen and progesterone, produced in much larger quantities in younger women.

Breast cancer survivors of all ages have similar concerns, such as: *Will I survive this? What will treatment be like? Will I have long-term side effects? Will I still look attractive to my partner? Will I still look attractive to myself?*

But younger women may have to juggle surgeries, chemotherapy, and radiation with raising children or launching a demanding career. Younger women—especially those who have not yet found a life partner—are especially concerned about how cancer will affect their self-image, sex life, and odds of finding a mate. They fear treatments may impair their fertility, robbing them of the opportunity to bear children. They worry about the amount of hormones their bodies are still producing and wonder how much this increases their risk of recurrence.

Most of all, younger women worry that their lives will end decades too soon. Five-year survival rates are not reassuring enough when you're hoping for another 30, 40, or 50+ years of cancer-free survival.

The background color of the *YSC* home page is hot-pink fuchsia, the same shade as the puffy taffeta dresses the bridesmaids wore at my wedding. The *YSC* site features a bulletin board with discussions about treatment, reconstruction, metastatic disease, early menopause, fertility after treatment, and sexuality. The posts are heartfelt, honest, funny, angry, and irreverent. I start to pretend we're a smart-aleck girl gang like the "Pink Ladies" in *Grease*. Some of the women have the caustic wit and skepticism of Stockard Channing's Rizzo, while others have the cheery and encouraging tone of Didi Conn's Frenchy. Occasionally, a flame war breaks out and feelings get singed, but underneath is true caring and compassion.

My *YSC* sisters form special groups based on timelines for surgeries and treatment, walking through Cancerland together. Kind and courageous women post photos on the reconstruction bulletin board, so that newly-diagnosed sisters will know what to expect when they look in the mirror. Veteran *YSC* sisters, years past treatment, check back in to celebrate

---

DS

Divine Secret: Seek out your pink tribe, the group that feels right to you.

All breast cancer survivors are Ta-Ta Sisters, but just like all families, sometimes you'll feel closer to one sister than another. Find the support group that feels right for you. I cannot over-emphasize how helpful it is to make this connection.

survivorship milestones and offer encouragement.

Sometimes, my *YSC* sisters vent about clueless or boneheaded remarks others make. They share details, such as chemotherapy regimens and reconstruction choices. Friends and family want to be supportive, but only another Pink Sister fully understands the pervasive fear of the unknown, the roller-coaster of staging and treatment, the seemingly endless time required for physical and psychological healing.

My *YSC* sisters *know* how cancer changes you in physical and invisible ways.

Resources:

Check with your hospital for information about local breast cancer support groups. If there's not a meeting close or convenient enough to attend, consider joining an online community, where you can log on anytime. Spend a little time reading their discussion boards so you can find the right fit.

For support, information, and conversation, check out:

• youngsurvival.org—YSC focuses on the needs of women diagnosed in their 20s, 30s, and 40s.

• metavivor.org—METAvivor offers support to those diagnosed with metastatic (Stage IV) breast cancer.

• sharsheret.org—Sharsheret provides support to young Jewish women.

• sistersnetworkinc.org—Sisters Network Inc. is a national organization of African American survivors.

• tnbcfoundation.org—The Triple Negative Breast Cancer Foundation assists women with a subtype of cancer unresponsive to estrogen, progesterone, and HER/2 receptors.

• breastcancer.org—This non-profit helps women understand the complex medical and personal information about breast cancer so they can make the best decision for their lives.

♡ 13

Where's my Booby Prize?

In the days prior to my appointment, I google-stalk the plastic surgeon, finding his impressive medical credentials. Bonus points—he's a bona fide artist with illustrations in medical textbooks. He's also a humanitarian, volunteering on overseas medical missions to correct the cleft palates of needy children, so I put a photo in my purse of Cara Li, a baby girl in our Adoption Travel Group who received this surgery. I have high hopes for my appointment!

As Ryan and I walk into the plastic surgery practice, I realize we've entered an alternate universe. Expecting typical waiting-room decor—chairs with washable upholstery, industrial gray carpet, wrinkled, outdated *Time* magazines— I'm stunned by the leather sofas, brocade draperies, and gilt-framed oil paintings. This place looks like the Ritz-Carlton lobby!

Behind the polished, intricately carved rosewood desk, attractive receptionists with perky boobs and pouty collagen lips register patients. *Must be an employee discount.* One of them hands me a beeper. I suppose this is done in an effort to ensure privacy—after all, some society doyennes will never admit to having any "work" done—but the gadget reminds me of waiting for my table at Macaroni Grill.

I take a seat next to my husband. While he studies his Blackberry, I flip through copies of *Town & Country*, *Vanity Fair*, and *Vogue* fanned across the table, admiring photographs of shoes that would cost me the equivalent of one month's mortgage. Peeking out from behind my magazine, I observe the other patients, wondering why they're here. *Did the young woman in that baggy sweatshirt have a breast augmentation or reduction? Does the older lady with the gold bangles and designer handbag want a facelift?*

Before long, my beeper goes off, so we follow yet another attractive female to a different, slightly more clinical waiting room. There must be some unspoken policy about not hiring any homely employees! After filling out paperwork, we're escorted past an Asian-themed atrium to an exam room, where I'm instructed to change into a gown. Minutes later, the surgeon walks in. Rather young, with a serious, modest demeanor, he has the glossy raven hair and swarthy complexion of a Bollywood actor.

"Nice to meet you," I say. "I've heard about your humanitarian work." I reach into my purse for Cara Li's photo.

"Yes, yes, I am leaving on another trip in a few months," he replies, his forehead crinkling in sincerity.

"Our daughter was born in China. This little girl was in our adoption group." I hand him the photo. "After surgery, she was matched with a wonderful family."

He glances at the picture and nods.

"If her cleft palate hadn't been repaired," I add, "she would've been categorized as special needs, decreasing her chances of being matched."

"Yes, yes," he replies, the lilt in his voice increasing. *Guess he's not one for chit-chat.*

I explain that I'm considering a mastectomy and want to know my options.

"Her surgeon is recommending lumpectomy, but she's not sure," Ryan adds.

"Do you have photos of previous patients I can see?"

"No, no, I haven't put an album together yet. The photos are all in my computer."

This seems odd. I'd thought all plastic surgeons had portfolios. "I'd really like to see some reconstructions you've done."

"You can make an appointment to come back another time. My nurse will find some photos for you to view." His forehead scrunches, as if he's puzzled by my request. I immediately dub him Dr. Quizzical.

"Okay…"

"Most breast reconstruction at this office is done using implants."

I suppress a sigh. Despite Zen-like decorative touches, this exam room is not giving me any good Foob Feng Shui. "I'm not keen on implants." I've seen too many weird tabloid photos of skeletal celebrities with unnatural, disproportionate globes attached to their chests.

"Fake is okay by me," Ryan adds. "I think you'd look good with implants."

I give my husband the evil eye, telegraphing that I'm not seeking his opinion at the moment. "What about tissue-transfer reconstruction, such as DIEP or muscle-sparing TRAM?" What I've read about DIEP (Deep Inferior Epigastric Perforator) sounds especially appealing, because none of your abdominal muscles are removed, just skin, tissue, fat, and blood vessels, giving you a complimentary tummy tuck.

"No one in town does DIEP," Dr. Quizzical replies.

I slump, weighed down by the disappointing news.

"You have to be specially trained. It is a complicated micro-surgery where tiny blood vessels are grafted together."

He explains that DIEP surgery may take as long as six to eight hours for a single reconstruction and over twelve for a bilateral. Then the patient must remain in the hospital for at least a week, with the room temperature so elevated it feels like a sauna. Nurses examine the new tissue transfer by ultrasound around the clock for signs of failure.

"I would love to do it sometime but we are not equipped. It's possible there is someone qualified at Chapel Hill or Duke. If not, you would need to travel to one of the specialized DIEP surgical centers in New Orleans or New York."

I'm not totally surprised, but can't help feeling disappointed. Following the breast reconstruction chat on the *YSC* site, I've read posts of women raving about their DIEP results. Admittedly, though, most had to travel long distances and fight with their insurers to authorize the procedure. So I ask about another procedure, Transverse Rectus Abdominal Muscle Flap, aka TRAM.

"What about muscle-sparing TRAM? I've read it requires only a tiny bit of muscle."

"Yes, I could do that." Dr. Quzzical frowns and shakes his head. "While not as complicated as DIEP, TRAM is still a lengthy surgery. You'd have a long hospital stay and extended recovery time."

Yeah, but a week in the hospital watching cable TV doesn't seem too bad a price to pay. Not if I could end up with a flat stomach and a nice rack.

"It is impossible to know before surgery whether the muscle-sparing variant of the procedure would work for you. I must decide in the operating room. It all depends on your anatomy."

I'm starting to frown now, too.

"Also, there is the risk of serious complications. If we take muscle, then you will lose abdominal strength. You will find it difficult, maybe impossible, to do sit-ups."

"I could live with that." If I can get a flat tummy with surgery, then who cares whether I can do sit-ups?

"There are many things you do using your abdominal muscles," he warns. "Lifting heavy objects, getting out of bed, even coughing."

My mind races as I think of a work-around. *I can get Ryan or the boys to move furniture and carry heavy boxes. Maybe I can roll out of bed, using my arms and legs for leverage.*

"You will be more prone to back problems and hernias."

My eyes well with tears.

"The important thing is to rid your body of cancer," the doctor reminds me.

"He's right," Ryan adds.

Dr. Quizzical hands me a tissue. I'm strategizing how to squeeze lemonade from a crummy cancer lemon, but it sounds like he's trying to talk me out of TRAM reconstruction, too.

"Let's take a look at you." He calls in a nurse to assist. She's holding a camera.

Embarrassed, I open my hospital gown. At this point, between the original mammography tech, diagnostic tech, radiologists, biopsy technicians, Rock Star Surgeon, and his staff, at least a dozen people have seen my bare breasts in the last few weeks. You'd think I'd feel less awkward by this point.

Dr. Quizzical measures different dimensions of my breasts and abdomen.

"You don't have enough tissue for a bilateral TRAM reconstruction," he says. "I would recommend only doing the one breast."

Is he kidding? My worst figure flaw has always been my abundant belly. Even in my teens and early 20s, I always had extra tummy fat. I remember sprawling across the bed in my college dorm so I could zip up my Gloria Vanderbilt jeans before heading out to a frat party.

"Please allow me to take some photos."

Dr. Quizzical has me face the camera, then turn sideways. I feel awkward and shy. *If somebody is pointing a camera at my breasts, why can't it be the* Girls Gone Wild *photographer?* At least I could down a few margaritas in Cozumel beforehand. Alas, there's not much demand for DVDs of middle-aged soccer moms lifting their shirts.

"As I said earlier, most of the reconstructions at this office are done with implants."

I get a mental vision of Pamela Anderson, top-heavy and tattooed. "I don't know. I don't want to look unnatural. But I have heard a lot of women choose immediate reconstruction with implants."

"You must realize 'immediate reconstruction' is a misnomer," he explains. "I would place two expanders beneath your chest muscles. You would then come to the office every week or two. The expanders are filled with saline water until the skin and underlying muscle are adequately stretched. Then, we return to the operating room to exchange the expander for the implant. Following that, there are additional surgeries to make revisions and add nipples. The entire process can take 12 to 18 months."

Why can't there be a truly quick and easy option?

"Also, I cannot tell you what size you will be after the implants."

"What do you mean?" *This doesn't make sense.*

"The largest implant is 800cc. I don't know if that's big enough. Most of the time we are augmenting breast tissue already there, but after cancer that tissue has been removed."

"Couldn't we aim for a C cup, not too big and not too small?" My jaw is starting to clench.

"You could go smaller, but you may not like the results. You will have extra skin remaining."

"Couldn't that be removed?"

"Yes, but that means even more scars."

I can deal with scars, I think. I just want a pair of moderately-sized breasts that look normal underneath my clothes.

"A few recent patients—the large-breasted ones—have not been pleased by their outcomes."

Exasperated, I sigh and don't even try to hide my eye roll. Sure, everyone jokes about doctors with huge egos, but isn't a certain confidence mandatory? I mean, who wants to go under the knife of an indecisive or hesitant surgeon? "I'm not sure what to do."

"I can do the TRAM if you wish. You should have enough tissue for one breast. We could reduce and lift the other."

Tears cloud my eyes again. At first, it sounded like he was steering me away from a tissue-transfer procedure. Now he's saying he'll do it if I want? This seems weird. Should I choose an operation he's advising against? "A few minutes ago, you said TRAM wouldn't be a good idea."

"It is your choice. I can do whichever operation you prefer."

I glance at Ryan, wondering if he's feeling as confused as I am. "I-I-I don't know." I reach for another tissue. "I guess I'll have to think about things. Maybe I should give some more thought to implants."

Divine Secret: Sometimes everything seems incredibly complicated.

You'll have to make a number of tough decisions—more than you ever realized. Answers won't always come easily, so keep investigating the pros and cons until you get the information you need.

"Let me know your decision. My nurse will book the operating room for a date and time agreeable with your breast surgeon." Dr. Quizzical bids us goodbye and leaves the room.

Feeling downcast and more perplexed than before the appointment, I look at Ryan.

He gives me a hug. "It's okay. Getting rid of the cancer is what's important."

I had been confident that after visiting the plastic surgeon, I would learn how—unlike a female Humpty-Dumpty—I could be put back together again, but it isn't going to be easy.

Asking the Big Guy for a Little Help

Ryan drops me off at home and heads to his office. Mom has been staying at our house to help while we've been tied up with doctor appointments. The kids are playing with friends, so we have a quiet moment to talk.

"What did the plastic surgeon say?"

"Nothing I wanted to hear." I slump into a chair. "I don't know what to think. I feel really confused."

She hands me a cup of tea and joins me at the kitchen table. "Did you like him?"

"He was very formal, but nice enough. Mostly, I didn't like what he said." I sigh and take a sip of tea. "He told me I don't have enough stomach flab for bilateral reconstruction. Can you believe that?"

"What did he recommend?"

"I think he's steering me toward implants, because he kept talking about all the possible side effects and complications from tissue transfer. Like back problems and not being able to lift heavy items."

"You have to consider those things. You'll want to pick up your grandchildren someday."

"But I was really counting on that free tummy tuck! Why can't I get at least one good thing out of this lousy experience?"

"Joanna, focus!" Mom replies, her voice suddenly sharp. "You have CANCER. Forget about the stupid tummy tuck. Watch what you eat and go to the gym or, if it really bothers you, get a tummy tuck sometime in the future."

"You're right," I admit. "Cancer is my deadly enemy, not stomach flab."

Looks like I might have to kiss the free tummy tuck goodbye, unless I can redeem surplus frequent flier miles for it, like you can for a panini grill or magazine subscriptions.

Mom's comment snaps me back to reality. I've kept myself busy fretting over reconstruction options as a way to avoid thinking about the cancer. Kind of like cleaning the oven while the house is burning down.

But now I turn the focus to the main issue: chances are quite good that my breast cancer is early-stage and very treatable. But we won't know for certain until after surgery, not before the tumor is removed and the surrounding tissue and lymph nodes are examined and tested. Then there's the worry that a few rogue cancer cells have floated into other parts of my body and could raise their ugly heads sometime in the future.

I've got to push aside my reconstruction concerns and prepare to fight this beast however possible. Alex, Nick, and Larissa need me! I decide that, at every decision, I'll take the option that will maximize my odds of long-term, recurrence-free survival.

~

I log onto my computer and see that many of our travel group friends have sent warm messages of support. I click on my *CaringBridge* site and write a snarky update about the lavish waiting room at the plastic surgeon's office. My cancer blog might end up being a really cool thing. I can give people updates and share funny stories without having to repeat myself a million times or answer a multitude of questions.

It doesn't take long to figure out the next group of people

I should send my *CaringBridge* link to—our friends from church. Every week, members of our Sunday school class share concerns. I'd welcome their prayers on my behalf.

After Ryan and I relocated from Texas, it took a while to locate the right spiritual home. For the first few years, we attended a vibrant, growing church in a university town about 40 minutes away. The preacher at Collegiate Church was a brilliant speaker, delivering sermons every week that provoked reflection and discussion. However, because of the distance, it was hard to participate in weeknight activities and get acquainted with people.

Then we spent several years attending a lovely church in our town. The buildings and landscaping at Country Club Church were gorgeous, but with a distinctly upscale congregation, it didn't feel right either. While I can appreciate an elegant lifestyle, day-to-day I'm more comfortable with stainless steel than sterling silver. (And many times I'm totally cool with a plastic spork.)

My spiritual Goldilocks experiment ended when we found our just-right place at Down Home Church. Alex and Nick joke around, calling it our Redneck Church. They never miss a chance to point out the outline of a pocketknife or Skoal can in someone's back pocket. Many in the congregation have chosen helping professions, so there's a large contingent of firefighters, teachers, and nurses.

Down Home Church feels like a large and extended family, with a few cranky aunts and crazy uncles thrown into the mix. Lloyd, the senior pastor, and Barry, the associate pastor, are like yin and yang. Lloyd grew up in a Pentecostal household and sometimes his speech takes on a slightly hammy and theatrical vibe, like he's in a community theatre production of King Lear. His sermons are funny and riveting. Nobody falls asleep when he's talking. He's also struggled with serious health issues of his own in recent years and has great empathy for his parishioners.

In contrast to Lloyd's exuberant personality, Barry is cerebral and self-effacing, a braniac with a dry wit that sneaks up on you. His spouse, Marie, is completely unlike any stereotype you might hold about a preacher's wife. Feisty and funny, she is refreshingly tart rather than saccharine sweet. When Barry preaches, you can almost see him unraveling knotted theological questions, grappling with how to reconcile the flesh and the spirit, the present and the eternal. On the day we became full-fledged members of Down Home Church, every single parishioner shook our hands and welcomed our family.

Normally, I'm fairly independent and don't like asking others for help. I want to do things my own way. This carries over into my spiritual life, because although I believe in a Higher Power, I don't often like bothering Him. But cancer is a pretty big problem and not something I can resolve on my own.

I yearn for a sense of hopefulness to wrap around me like a warm, fuzzy blanket. I want to believe that Somebody out there in the universe hears little insignificant me over all the world's craziness and commotion. Sort of like when *Horton Hears a Who*.

"Hey, God," I whisper. "Forgive me for ignoring You lately. I'm sorry I haven't talked to You much."

My attempt at prayer feels strained and awkward, like making small talk on a blind date.

"Joanna, what's wrong?" Strangely, the voice in my head sounds more like Ryan Seacrest than Kirk Douglas.

"I've been diagnosed with breast cancer."

"I know. I've always known."

"Then why did You ask?"

"So you'd know I'm listening."

"Please help me through this," I plead.

I'm not sure exactly how I picture God or if He should really be envisioned as male, with a long beard and flowing robe. The term "Heavenly Father" has always left me flummoxed and annoyed since I didn't have a good relationship with my biological dad. I prefer to think of my Higher Power as a "Heavenly Grandpa." Sort of like my late Grandfather Windsor, a kind and steadfast man I still miss thirty years after his passing.

I take a deep breath, trying to feel God's embrace. A sweet and comforting feeling like when Grandfather Windsor took me for double-scoop ice cream cones. (*Yeah, even the most incompetent therapist could make a few assumptions about my food-equals-love issues. But maybe some days I just like to spend quality time with a bag of Oreos.*)

I've always yearned to know God and to feel His presence. I have vivid memories of a summer church camp I attended at age 10. Every night at chapel time, after a day filled with swimming and macramé classes, the pastor would call on children to recite Bible verses. If they had memorized the verses correctly, they'd win a colorful chalk drawing of that evening's topic. On the first night, the prize was a picture of Noah's Ark, illustrated with animal pairs and a rainbow in the sky. I raised my hand, hoping to be called upon, but was passed over.

The next evening, I'd rehearsed my assigned Bible verse in hopes of winning that evening's prize, a depiction of the Sermon on the Mount, where disciples handed out baskets of bread and fish on the hillside. But no matter how much I bounced up and down in my chair, flailing my arm, I was ignored.

That is, until the last night of church camp.

Once again, I'd diligently memorized my verse and was prepared to win. With a flourish, the pastor unrolled the canvas to reveal a picture of John the Baptist's decapitated head on a blood-splattered platter, his eyes all googly, his tongue lolling sideways.

I was aghast; the picture creeped me out! I remember thinking it was a strange thing to give a child. Yet all around me, fellow campers raised their hands and shouted "Ooh! Ooh!" hoping to be called upon.

The pastor pointed at me. "Young lady, can you recite tonight's Bible verse?"

"No," I lied, as my cheeks flushed in shame.

I knew I was probably in big trouble with God for being dishonest. But dang, John the Baptist's lifeless eyeballs would have haunted me if I'd taken that picture home.

In the years since, I've wrestled with questions of faith: of what I know, what I believe, what I hope. I take issue with all the religious groups who think they've figured it all out, who are egotistical enough to think they are the only ones spiritually correct. It seems that we humans spend an excessive amount of time worrying about whether we should be sprinkled or dunked, eat kosher foods or bacon cheeseburgers, wear magical underwear or Kabbalah bracelets. Frankly, I believe God loves everyone—Christian, Buddhist, Muslim, Jew—and probably has little patience for our petty religious squabbles.

Divine Secret: Ask yourself what you believe.

There's so much I can't possibly understand, but I do believe in a loving Higher Power. Consider how the religious teaching of your childhood, as well as your faith experiences as an adult, can be a source of comfort and reassurance.

I'm Not Completely Crazy

My stomach has been in knots for days. Rock Star Surgeon and Dr. Point Guard assure me I'm a great candidate for lumpectomy, but I still can't get comfortable with the idea. This is distressing because I think of myself as a fairly logical person. I've read more of the research explaining how—for patients meeting the criteria—survival rates are equivalent for mastectomy *or* lumpectomy plus radiation. I have faith in my doctors and respect their advice, but continue to feel uneasy.

There are good reasons to prefer lumpectomy. One is minimal disfigurement—maybe just a scar or divot—completely hidden in a bra or bathing suit. Also, it's usually done as an outpatient procedure, requiring neither an overnight hospital stay nor yucky surgical drains. A lumpectomy definitely offers a quicker, easier recovery.

If all goes well, Rock Star Surgeon would grant me permission to go on a long-planned cruise with Ryan's family. I'm already on the surgery schedule, so in a few weeks I could be recuperating on a lounge chair, martini glass of frozen pain-killer in hand.

Yet my mind turns in circles, questioning everything. *Is the little voice inside me nothing more than a manifestation of anxiety? Or is it an intuitive message I need to heed?*

At my computer, I log onto the *Young Survival Coalition* site. I post a message asking my Pink Sisters how they decided between mastectomy and lumpectomy.

Immediately, my *YSC* friends write replies. *Ta-Ta Sisters to the rescue!*

Some tell me that due to fear of future mammograms, they opted for mastectomy. Once you've received a cancer diagnosis, anything the least bit abnormal will be scrutinized. Others chose mastectomy because of a strong family history (with or without BRCA mutations, genetic traits indicating a higher likelihood of developing breast or ovarian cancer). Too many *YSC* Sisters have watched their grandmothers, mothers, aunts, sisters, and cousins battle this ugly disease. Worried about their future, they chose to dodge this bullet.

In contrast, other women offered this option chose lumpectomy, wanting to minimize cancer's effect on their appearance. Their breasts made them feel sexy and beautiful, and they didn't want that taken away. Also, they preferred the less radical surgery and recovery time.

I post my next question on the *YSC* website: *Did any of you regret your decision?* I scan their replies.

Almost every Pink Sister says she's comfortable with her choice and has no regrets.

As Rock Star Surgeon had explained, some of the women who'd had a lumpectomy needed one or more re-excisions. Several who'd had lumpectomies confessed a lingering fear of recurrence, relentlessly checking their breasts. But most were happy their breasts retained sensation and didn't need reconstruction.

Upon reflection, a few *YSC* gals felt they'd been too hasty in deciding on mastectomy, acting out of fear instead of carefully weighing their options. Many of the women relied on their doctors' advice to make their decisions. Most doctors look at the hard data—valid, reliable research gleaned over years of study—plus tumor size, aggressiveness, and family history, as well as how easily your breasts can be screened for future problems.

However, there's no way to quantify feelings.

I'm the one who must live with the results. I'll be the one looking in the mirror.

Ultimately, the decision is mine.

~

I'm scheduled for the breast MRI, a scan much more sensitive than a mammogram. It's used to determine the extent of DCIS (Stage 0, non-invasive cancer), which can be widespread, or for planning purposes prior to surgery. Breast MRIs are sometimes recommended for women with very dense breast tissue or who are considered high-risk.

The imaging center is in the basement of the large downtown hospital where Rock Star Surgeon practices. After a few tense minutes in the lobby, the MRI technician calls my name and leads me to the changing area. I undress, remove all jewelry, and don yet another flimsy hospital gown.

She escorts me to an enormous tunnel-like contraption. Unlike many brightly-fluorescent exam rooms, the space is as dim as a cavern. They could really use a few aromatherapy candles to soften the cold, clinical edge.

"I'll start your IV line. We need to take some pictures with contrast."

I wince as the MRI tech searches for a vein, plunging the needle into my arm.

She positions me on a platform, facing down, my breasts hanging through cut-outs, my forehead held in place by a spongy headrest. With the push of a button, I slide into the tunnel while she steps into the anti-radioactive protected area and turns on a loudspeaker.

"Hold very still."

I concentrate on not moving as the MRI makes loud thumping noises. I try to imagine a beach with the seagulls flying overhead, the waves crashing. *But I can't see it!* Then I try to imagine a lovely waterfall in the mountains, birds singing and water rushing. *Nada!* Anything to block out the ominous humming and clanging.

The MRI tech emerges from the glassed-in control room. "Good job. Now we need to take some with contrast." She holds up the syringe of dye that will spread throughout my body, lighting up trouble spots and suspicious areas. "You may feel a flushing sensation."

She injects the dye into my IV. A warm, tingly feeling spreads throughout my body. I'm dizzy, not sure if it's from the IV agent or anxiety.

"We're about halfway through." She repositions me on the platform and adjusts the foam headrest. Sliding back into the machine, I try to hold still and ignore the noise.

"All done." She helps me up from the table and removes the IV line.

"When will I get results?"

"Probably in a few days. The radiologist will send a report to your doctor. Then your doctor will contact you."

That's not soon enough! I'm desperate for information, for reassurance, for direction. "Could I talk to the radiologist, please?"

"The radiologists don't usually discuss results with patients."

"Could you make an exception? Just this once?"

The nurse bites her lip and looks at her clipboard.

"Please, I'm having a hard time," I confide, assuming a pitiful, beseeching expression. "My surgeon is recommending a lumpectomy, but I'm not sure. I really need to talk to the radiologist."

She sighs, recognizing that it would take a uniformed security officer to drag me out of there. "Okay, we'll see what he says."

We walk down the hall to an office to find the radiologist staring at his computer screen, scrutinizing splotches of red, blue, and green across a black and gray background. With his wire-framed glasses, mustache, curly hair, and a slightly nebbish manner, he resembles Gabe Kaplan's "Mr. Kotter" character.

He looks up, surprised by our interruption.

"Hi," I say. "Sorry to bother you." I give him a brief summary, explaining my dilemma.

Reluctant Radiologist fidgets in his chair, frowning. "I don't usually discuss results with patients. My report will go to your surgeon."

Maybe he prefers looking at X-rays over interacting with actual people, but I'm determined. "Please, I'm so confused right now. I could really use your opinion." I mimic Larissa's plaintive begging-for-candy expression, hoping it makes me look desperate but not demented.

"I'm going to be tied up for hours, reviewing all of today's test results, including yours."

"That's okay. I can wait."

Reluctant Radiologist sighs and massages his forehead, realizing I'm a headache that won't go away. "All right. Come back at 4 p.m."

∼

I have hours to spare, so I decide to spend the time downtown. People stroll along the sidewalks to appointments or lunch meetings. After grabbing a bite to eat, I head to the library, where I scan cancer reference books in a futile attempt at finding an answer.

Discouraged, I find a deserted area in the stacks, where my voice won't be a distraction, and call my gynecologist's office. I tell the receptionist why I'm calling, and she forwards me to his extension.

"Hello."

Simply hearing Calming Gynecologist's voice takes the edge off my nerves.

"Hi, thanks for taking my call," I answer. "Remember me? Age 45, just diagnosed with breast cancer."

"Yes, of course. How are you?"

"Not great," I tell him. "I have to decide between lumpectomy and mastectomy, but I'm very confused. I had the breast MRI this morning and am waiting for results."

"Hmm," he says. "Call me old-fashioned, but in my opinion, your first shot is your best shot in getting rid of the cancer."

"You'd advise a mastectomy?"

"Oncology is not my area of expertise. Maybe the breast MRI will help you decide. But, yes, I'd choose the more aggressive surgery. I've had patients your age who've battled breast cancer several times. You want to minimize the chance of that happening."

"Thank you," I say. "I appreciate your honesty."

"Good luck to you," Calming Gynecologist replies. "Call me anytime."

~

Time drags into the mid-afternoon. I return to the imaging center, watch the clock, and flip through magazines. I wonder how many women in this reception area have been diagnosed with breast cancer.

Finally, Reluctant Radiologist appears and ushers me into a small conference room.

"Thanks for agreeing to meet with me," I tell him. "I know it's not the norm."

"It's not something I usually do," he concurs, handing me several glossy pages that show the gray and black background of my breast tissue, blotched with green, blue, and red.

"See this area?" He points to a large green splotch. "That is the tumor that was biopsied."

At my diagnostic mammogram, I saw what looked like a single drop of white paint. The green area he's indicating on the MRI results is larger, more like a paintball splatter.

What does this mean? Maybe the tumor is not so tiny, after all?

He points to a second splotch. "I'm concerned about this." His face is solemn yet empathetic. "This area looks very suspicious. There's no way to know for certain without a biopsy, but based on my experience, I'd guess it's malignant as well."

*What? I have **two** tumors?*

No wonder I've felt confused and distraught. I remember the stereotactic biopsy, where I tried to convince Snippy Nurse and Kindly Doctor that they were looking in the wrong area.

I was right all along! They *were* looking in a different location than the one scrutinized at my diagnostic mammogram.

"I do have some encouraging news," Reluctant Radiologist adds. "Based on these scans, I don't see signs of lymph node involvement." He explains that I won't know for sure until after the sentinel node biopsy and pathology reports, but he's pleased that no nodes were lit up on his computer screen.

I'm relieved to hear this, but worry how multiple malignancies will affect my odds. *Does this change my staging? My prognosis?*

"Could I have a copy of these?"

He looks uncertain for a moment, but then agrees and steps out to make a copy.

Minutes later, he hands me several print-outs.

"I appreciate your willingness to talk with me." I explain that I had not felt good about scheduling a lumpectomy despite Rock Star Surgeon's recommendation.

"He's an excellent surgeon, one of the best," Reluctant Radiologist says. "I know he prefers breast-conserving surgery when possible. He's a leader in cutting-edge procedures."

The bespectacled doctor glances down at the scans and then looks up at me. "But if you were my wife or daughter, I'd want you to have a mastectomy."

I have my answer. It all makes sense now. There was a reason for my ambivalence. "Thank you!"

Reluctant Radiologist must think I'm nuts, because suddenly I'm acting giddy, like I'm going to hug him or something.

"Good luck," he says, backing out of the conference room, a cautious look on his face. "I'll tell your surgeon about our conversation."

~

I get in my minivan and call Ryan. "Guess what? There are *two* tumors!"

He doesn't respond immediately, puzzled by my jubilant tone. No woman in her right mind would be happy to learn of more than one tumor. Yet I feel vindicated; my intuition had been right all along.

Divine Secret: Don't ignore that little voice inside you.

You usually make the best decisions when your intellect and your gut feelings are in harmony. I kept feeling an inner uneasiness I couldn't chalk up to anxiety. Ta-Ta Sisters, you need hard data to make decisions, but don't overlook or dismiss the importance of intuition.

Bumps in the Road

The next morning, I get a call from Rock Star Surgeon's office.

"Hi, Joanna," says Caring Nurse. "How are you?"

"I'm okay. I had my breast MRI yesterday."

"So I heard," she answers. "We saw the report this morning. Would you like me to set up an appointment to discuss the results?"

"Yes, thanks," I reply. "I, um, talked to the radiologist. He said it looked like there may be a second tumor, so I'm definitely thinking mastectomy."

"Yes, the radiologist mentioned your conversation in his report." Calm and pleasant, her voice betrays no sign of irritation that I circumvented the normal channels for medical feedback. I ask if she knows Rock Star Surgeon's reaction to the MRI.

"I'm looking at your chart right now, and I see 'mastectomy' written across the top and underlined."

"Okay, we're on the same page." I'm strangely relieved there was a valid reason behind my confusion. I'm not a superstitious person, but I'll accept that sometimes we have an inner wisdom that can't be explained.

"We did get your test results. And you are highly estrogen and progesterone positive, which means you can benefit from the adjuvant therapy drugs, like tamoxifen."

"Thanks! I'm glad to finally know for certain."

Caring Nurse schedules an appointment with Rock Star Surgeon. I jot the date and time down in my pocket calendar.

"Take care," she says. "And call me if you have any questions or want to talk before you come in."

~

Once again, I'm at the computer, googling information about multi-focal (in the same quadrant) and multi-centric (in different quadrants) breast cancer. What does having two separate tumors mean in terms of my staging and treatment? Could cancer be lurking in my lymph nodes, even though Reluctant Radiologist said they looked good? Does this change my odds?

Too impatient to wait for answers at my next appointment, I stare at the computer screen, trying to decipher the statistics and terminology. According to current treatment guidelines from the National Cancer Institute (NCI), when there are multiple breast malignancies, the size of the largest tumor *alone* determines staging. Therefore, my prognosis may not change despite a second malignancy. *Good news!*

However, not every oncologist agrees. Scattered across the Internet, I find studies where the authors suggest staging and treatment should be based on total tumor load—the sum size of all invasive cancers in the breast.

Who's right? What should I believe?

Conflicting opinions are unsettling; I need some emergency carbs and mindless distraction.

Opening the fridge, I break off a few pieces of chocolate chip cookie dough. Not bothering to put them in the oven, I carry them upstairs and turn on the TV.

~

The next day, after taking Larissa to preschool camp, I run

into Will, Hannah's husband. As a nurse anesthetist, he's seen plenty of surgeries, so I decide to ask questions even if it feels awkward.

"Hey, Will," I say. "I'd like your opinion."

"Sure."

Underneath his country-boy drawl, Will has a razor-sharp intellect. He's usually quiet, but becomes animated when discussing his work.

"I know you've seen a fair amount of breast reconstruction. What do you think of TRAM—where they create a fake boob out of abdominal tissue? Does it end up looking natural?"

"I've seen some turn out nice. It's a long operation though."

"Yeah, I've heard. What's your opinion on breast implants?"

A mom walking through the parking lot overhears and gives me a strange look. Maybe it's inappropriate to talk about my boobs in the preschool parking lot, but desperate times call for desperate measures.

"From the surgeries I've seen," he says, "those implants look pretty damn good."

"Really?"

"Yeah," he says, trying to suppress a grin. "I've seen some nice results."

"That's great to hear! I'm looking at all my options."

"Let me know your surgery date," he says. "I'll check the schedule and see who's working in the OR that day. Make sure they take good care of you."

"Thanks!"

It would be weird having Will responsible for my anesthesia. I'd feel awkward eating pizza with him at a Chuck E. Cheese birthday party after he'd seen me splayed out on the operating table. But I'm glad he'll tell his co-workers to watch over me.

∼

There are about a zillion things I need to get done while Larissa is at camp, but instead I'm clutching the remote. I'm not usually into TV—I'd much rather read—but lately it's served as electronic Prozac for my anxiety.

I click the remote past *CNN Headline News* and *Law & Order* reruns when suddenly I come across *The Girls Next Door*, a salacious "reality" show about life at the Playboy mansion with Hugh Hefner and his three bleached blonde, boobalicious girlfriends.

If I've been seeking validation for breast implants, then this is the mother lode! Mortified yet mesmerized, I can't stop staring at the girls. Holly, Bridget, and Kendra cavort topless in the pool, pose for photo shoots, and watch classic movies with a wrinkly, shuffling Hef. It's like an X-rated sorority house with a senior citizens wing. I'll admit the blonde trio looks good, albeit a bit too amply endowed for my taste. Implants following expanders *are* the most popular breast reconstruction technique. Maybe I'd look okay even if I'll never be mistaken for Barbie Benton or any other aging Playmate. Let's just get this done!

Picking up the phone, I call Rock Star Surgeon's office and ask to speak to Surgery Scheduler.

"I've made some decisions," I tell her. "Thought you'd like a heads up. I know it's difficult coordinating multiple surgeons and booking operating rooms."

"Okay." She sounds hesitant, unsure.

But I'm just being pro-active, right? Not control-freaky?

"Let's plan for a bilateral mastectomy with immediate reconstruction using expanders." I mention that my oncologist has suggested a port (a semi-permanent valve used to deliver chemotherapy meds) be inserted at the same time.

Maybe I'm seriously speaking out of turn. But what do I have to lose, aside from annoying them? After all, Dr. Quizzical, the ambivalent plastic surgeon, is leaving for another mission trip in six weeks and logistics can be complicated. Furthermore, I'm growing crazier every day my body continues to harbor this cancer. It's a ticking time bomb that must be defused.

~

We call Dianne, Ryan's oldest sister, and give her an update. Maybe after a lumpectomy I would be able to go on the cruise, but mastectomy is going to require a longer recuperation.

"I'm sorry you're going through this," my sister-in-law says.

"Having cancer is bad enough," I joke, "but missing a vacation? That really stinks!"

"Why don't you send the kids with us? I'll watch out for them."

I'm touched by her offer because our boys can be a handful. Ryan's sisters and their families are good-hearted people who really love their nieces and nephews.

"That's so sweet, Dianne, but they could be a hassle."

"It's no problem," she reassures me. "There will be plenty of us onboard to keep tabs on Alex and Nick. And you'll need a few days of peace and quiet."

Hmm. Larissa is too little to go without us, but the boys could visit me in the hospital after my surgery before leaving. They'd enjoy spending time with family and have fun on the ship.

~

I'm so damned tired of thinking about cancer, reading about cancer, talking about cancer. And I haven't even undergone surgery—the very first step. I want my normal life back.

The phone rings; it's Rock Star Surgeon. "I hear you've had some interesting conversations lately."

"Yes," I confess. "I kind of badgered the radiologist."

"Then you understand why I'm no longer recommending lumpectomy? I'd have to remove too much tissue. You'll need the mastectomy."

"Yes, and your nurse talked with me, too."

"I also heard you've talked with my surgery scheduler." His tone is pleasant, yet I hear tension underneath. "I know you'll be coming back for a pre-op appointment, but there are a few things we need to discuss."

"Okay."

"I don't want to do a bilateral right now. Let's take care of the cancer side first. And I'd prefer for you to do delayed reconstruction."

"Why?" I know Rock Star Surgeon likes to do breast-conserving surgeries whenever possible. That he's reluctant to perform a prophylactic mastectomy without strong reasons. *But why is he suggesting I put off reconstruction? Is he more concerned about the blotchy green splashes on my breast MRI than he's letting on?*

"A lot of patients have immediate reconstruction, and everything turns out fine. But I'm concerned about possible healing issues. You can't have chemotherapy until you've recovered from surgery. Any time there's an expander or any foreign object in your body, you increase the risk of infection."

"I was hoping to speed things up. Put cancer behind me."

Rock Star Surgeon sighs. I'm not his favorite patient at the moment. "I want you to reconsider the prophylactic surgery. Once I remove your unaffected breast, I can't put it back."

"I know. But I don't think I'd have regrets."

"Maybe not. But my main concern is that you might develop an infection on the non-cancer side, delaying chemo," he explains. "One of my colleagues has a patient with some positive lymph nodes. Her surgery was three months ago, but she's unable to start chemo because of healing issues on the *prophylactic* side."

I try to process what he's saying. I dread being lopsided, needing a prosthetic breast, facing multiple surgeries.

"There's always a ten to fifteen percent risk of infection after surgery," he continues. "It would be a shame to delay treatment because of healing issues. Let's deal with the cancer first."

Divine Secret: Realize that there are no shortcuts.

Your journey may take unexpected twists and turns or have frustrating setbacks and delays. It's an arduous, exhausting slog. Sometimes even the best plans go awry. Accept that you may face a long and circuitous path.

Rock Star Surgeon has a point. I want to tell this frigging cancer what to do, not let it boss me around. But I sought out a highly-regarded oncology surgeon, so I guess I should listen to his advice.

"Okay," I agree. "What do you think about the second tumor? Will this affect my prognosis?"

"I don't think so. Staging is done based on the size of the largest tumor."

I know that's the official party line, although there's some debate. Still, it's reassuring to hear him say so. "Would you want to install a port?"

"No," Rock Star Surgeon replies. "We don't know for certain you'll need chemotherapy. Let's not increase the risk of infection by adding other procedures."

Dang, it's going to be a long and bumpy road. Multiple surgeries, possible chemotherapy or radiation, then reconstruction. It could be nearly two years before I'm finished and can escape Cancerland.

17

With a Little Help from My Friends

L arissa and I attend a pool party with local families who've adopted daughters from China. We're celebrating the summer return of our friend Jessica and her family.

Jessica and I first met while waiting for our referrals, that magic moment when you get a phone call or a FedEx package with information and photos of your child. Though we never crossed paths in China, our adoption trips overlapped, with Jessica and her husband Steve leaving to get Sosie one week before we travelled to meet Larissa. Upon our return, we scheduled play dates and sought out other moms and babies to join us.

Jessica's family has spent the past year in Shanghai on an overseas work assignment. While there, they've been learning to speak Cantonese and gaining a deeper understanding of their daughter's birthplace. All the moms are eager to hear Jessica's stories.

Today, we've ordered pizza; the moms chat, our children splash in the water. I'm in the pool watching Larissa float on her inflatable water wings. My friend Tessa is nearby, keeping a close eye on her son and daughter.

"So," she asks. "What are you and the kids doing these last few weeks of summer?"

I hesitate for a minute, thinking of typical activities, not wanting to bring up the "C" word.

"Back-to-school shopping, I guess. Alex and Nick are going on a cruise with Ryan's family."

"Just the boys? Why aren't you all going?"

I mentally kick myself for bringing up the trip. *Dang.* The party's been great, catching up and hearing about Jessica's adventures in China. I don't want any gloomy clouds overshadowing the fun.

However, I'm fairly close to Tessa, and she's dealt with serious medical challenges, spending months at the hospital after her adorable red-headed son was born prematurely. I decide to confide in her.

"I can't go." I move closer, lessening the chance someone will overhear. "I'm having surgery. A mastectomy."

My stomach feels hollow every time I say the word.

"What?" Tessa's eyes widen.

"I've been diagnosed with breast cancer."

"Oh, no!" her forehead crinkles; she moves closer to me. "Hon, I am so sorry! Why didn't you tell us?"

"I don't want to spoil the fun." I glance at the kids jumping in the water, the moms laughing. "We haven't told many people yet."

"What can I do to help? You know we're here for you."

"Thanks," I answer, nodding in appreciation. Tessa is one of the most tender-hearted, caring people I know. Extremely bright and super-organized, she underestimates her talents. I sometimes joke she ought to be CEO of a Fortune 500 company—those Wharton MBAs in pinstripe suits have nothing on her.

I'm ambivalent about accepting help. But it could make a difficult time easier. "I know people will bring food," I say. "Would you coordinate the meal schedule?"

"Of course! But, Joanna," she urges, "you need to tell everyone."

"I know. But not now. Later today."

I can't bring myself to say anything at the pool party. It was easier to tell my Adoption Travel Group since we're spread across the country. And it wasn't too hard to disclose to church friends since a key part of Sunday School time is sharing concerns and requesting prayers. But the more people who know, the more real the cancer becomes. However, Tessa's right—I don't need to do this on my own.

~

Returning home, I type up an e-mail message to the local China playgroup moms and hit "send." *There!* Another social circle notified. Reclining on the couch, I brainstorm strategies for whacking cancer upside the head with my metaphorical Mary Poppins umbrella.

I think about a recent message posted on the *YSC* bulletin board by a wise Pink Sister: "When you accept help, you are helping the giver, too." She's right; friends and family want concrete ways to express their love, so by embracing their covered dishes, you're giving them a gift, allowing them to play an active role in the healing process. This sage Pink Sister explains that the food nurtures not only your body, but also your soul, promoting healing on multiple levels.

Okay! Bring on the macaroni tuna bake and the beef stroganoff. I will take her advice.

While I'm recovering, and possibly undergoing chemo or radiation, my energy levels will be depleted. The most important thing is being able to spend time with my kids. So, whenever someone asks if they can do something, I will say "Yes" and give them an assignment, such as going to the grocery store, driving me to an appointment, or taking over my carpool duties.

Since Tessa is so efficient, we won't end up with a freezer full of lasagnas in a single weekend. Liz and Hannah have offered to take me to coffee or lunch before every surgery or treatment for a friendly boost of caffeine and courage. Other friends are planning "dinner and movie" nights to give me something fun to anticipate during recovery. Also, Mom will be staying with us at times to keep the household running. Without a doubt, the house will be cleaner than when I'm in charge.

I take a deep breath. *Not done yet.*

My biggest concern is my children. I pick up the phone and call the parents of their closest friends. When I tell them about my health situation, they're shocked, but quickly offer to keep a watchful eye on Alex, Nick, and Larissa. I know they'll invite Larissa for play-dates or the boys to hang out, giving them an escape from the worry and anxiety at home.

Next, I call the counselors at the elementary, middle, and high schools. Each kid is moving up to a new school this year. I'd like Larissa to be assigned to a nurturing and sensitive kindergarten teacher. I want the boys' schools to understand our family is under stress and cut them a little slack if they forget an assignment or seem extra moody.

I finally hang up the phone, relieved to have these conversations done. Yakking about cancer is exhausting. I need a long nap and a large dose of therapeutic chocolate.

Divine Secret: Accept offers of help!

Many people will ask what they can do, but aren't sure what you need. Start brainstorming areas where you'd appreciate their help and how you could use their talents. Try to match volunteers with the tasks you'd think they'd do best. A free online service, lotsahelpinghands. org, offers a platform to organize your care-giving community. Friends and family can log onto your site, check the schedule to see what's needed, then sign up for tasks.

♡
18

I'm Such a Prude!

L ater that evening, I host book club. It's been a long day, but I'm looking forward to sipping a glass of wine with my book-loving pals. Numerous women have rotated in and out of book club over the past decade, all personable and interesting, but I'm particularly fond of the current members. Completely unpretentious, they're warm and honest about the challenges of parenting.

I've opened bottles of chardonnay and merlot. Warmed up mini-quiches and spinach dip. Placed a fruit tart on a pretty cake stand. I light a few candles, pushing away thoughts of cancer. I need to share my news, but I'll wait until right before everyone leaves. That way I can maximize the fun before turning into Debbie Downer.

But that doesn't happen.

Tessa arrives with a large gift bag. Moments later, Rebecca, the mom of one of Nick's friends, walks in with several bouquets of flowers from her garden. I'm touched by their thoughtfulness, yet slightly exasperated that the spotlight is on me.

"What's going on?" Simone asks.

"Tell them," urges Tessa.

"Do I have to?" I whine. "Can't we just drink wine and talk about the book?"

"Your friends need to know," Rebecca urges.

I take a deep breath. *Every time I talk about cancer, it makes it more real.* After making so many phone calls today, I'm tired of talking about it. But this is my reality. "I've, um, been diagnosed with breast cancer. And the doctors say I need a mastectomy."

My book club pals, with the exception of Tessa and Rebecca, all look shocked. Their mouths gape, foreheads crinkle. I fill them in: how the cancer was found during a routine mammogram and confirmed through a biopsy. Why I have to have a mastectomy rather than a lumpectomy. What my future treatments may be.

"We're all here for you," Patricia says.

Sarah nods. "What can we do to help?"

Tessa hands me the gift bag. I pull out a pink t-shirt and a black Sharpie pen. The shirt has a picture of a battleship with the words "I am a destroyer." On the back Tessa has written words of encouragement.

This brings tears to my eyes.

They pass the shirt around and everyone signs it with a personal message.

"Thank you so much," I say, blotting my eyes with a cocktail napkin. "I'll take it to the hospital for every surgery, every treatment."

~

The next day, I e-mail more friends and neighbors the link to my *CaringBridge* site. I include a brief update that cancer has been found in two places, so my surgical plans will be changing.

CaringBridge is a terrific way to communicate. I can let everyone know what's happening without repeating each story a zillion times. Within a few minutes of sending out the link, I start getting heartfelt, supportive e-mails.

~

A few nights later, Tessa arranges a group dinner at an upscale Chinese restaurant, inviting friends from my China playgroup and my book club, since she's involved in both. Entering the restaurant, I'm inundated with hugs and words of support.

"I'm so sorry," says Sue.

"You're so brave!" says Janet. "I love your blog!"

"Me, too," adds Tina. "Stay strong!"

"If humor's the best medicine, you're going to be just fine," insists Michelle.

I blush, accepting hugs until I've greeted everyone.

The hostess leads us to a large table. The woman beside me is a long-time survivor of ovarian cancer who later adopted two beautiful Chinese daughters. Ovarian is one of the stealthiest cancers, often showing only subtle symptoms. Frequently, the cancer has reached an advanced stage by the time it's discovered.

Teal Ribbon Mom is one of the lucky ones. She reaches over and touches my forearm. "Do you know if you'll be having chemotherapy?"

"Not for sure, but I think so. I want to do whatever I can to stop it from coming back."

"Joanna, I want to be your special chemo buddy. I can come to your house every day and do whatever you need. Make your meals, clean, whatever."

"Thank you," I reply, touched and a bit startled. "That's so sweet! Luckily, my mom is planning to stay with us."

"Listen, I know firsthand how difficult it will be," she says. "I'm serious. I can come to your house and take care of you. It'll give your mom a break. I really want to do this."

I like Teal Ribbon Mom and enjoy her company, but since we're not extremely close, I'm surprised at her insistence.

"Thanks so much," I say. "I'll definitely be seeking your advice. You'll be my personal cancer hotline!" I'm glad she'll welcome my questions. Even though Teal Ribbon Mom faced a different type of cancer, it's good to talk with someone who's been there, done that.

Since I'm not the designated driver, I order a second glass of chardonnay to accompany my ginger-glazed scallops.

"Joanna, do you mind if I ask you something?" Tessa asks.

"Go ahead."

I take another big gulp of wine. *Damn, this dinner is very nice, but I'd like to stop talking about cancer. Why can't we change the subject to global warming? Or home decorating ideas? Or funny pet stories?*

"Where else is the cancer? Your website mentioned that the cancer is in more than one place."

Oh, dear. Suddenly, I realize what I've done. I've created a big misunderstanding! Cancer, being such a grim and scary word, is often quickly—though not always accurately—interpreted as a harbinger of death.

I remember writing my latest *CaringBridge* update, purposely using vague language, too embarrassed to type the word "breast." After all, I grew up in a time when the word "pregnant" was considered vulgar; mothers-to-be were called "expectant." Even when talking to close friends, my tongue stumbles over the word "breast." I feel as awkward and naughty as a fifth-grade boy watching the animated sperm in the Jiminy Cricket sex education videos. How could I be such an uptight dinosaur, a downright prude, considering that every time I read a magazine, turn on the radio, or watch TV, my senses are bombarded by commercials for Viagra, penile enlargement, or feminine hygiene products?

I'm such an idiot! No wonder I've been getting so many heartfelt cards and e-mails.

"I'm really sorry," I explain. "I didn't make it

Divine Secret: Say the words without embarrassment.

Not long ago, cancers of the breast, uterus, cervix, and ovaries were alluded to as "female problems," something polite people shared only in whispers. But that era is over. Learn to say the words without blushing! Breast cancer is a terrible disease, but it's nothing to be embarrassed about. When you share health updates, be clear and specific to avoid misunderstandings.

clear. The tumors are both in my right breast. At this point, there's no indication that cancer has spread to other organs."

"That's great news!"

"Thank goodness!"

"I've been so worried. It's not good when you hear that cancer is in multiple places."

"I should have been more specific," I explain. "At this point, it looks like Stage I, caught early. But since there are two tumors, I definitely need a mastectomy rather than a lumpectomy. That's what I meant by a change in surgical plans."

Everyone at the table nods with relief and understanding.

"Okay," I joke. "I'm not at death's door. But will you bring me lasagna anyway?"

Sometimes You Need a Little Retail Therapy

The surgery countdown is on. I have a date on the calendar, less than two weeks away.

When the going gets tough, the tough go shopping. Mom and I head to the mall. Even during my rebellious teenaged years, we could always call a truce during retail therapy. Somehow, mother-daughter conflicts melted away in the presence of a clearance sign.

It'll take at least a month to recover from surgery, so I'm looking for pajamas to wear around the house. I want something comfortable, easy to put on and take off, and modest enough to wear around my adolescent sons.

I'm also looking for some drapey, oversized blouses to help camouflage the surgical drains—lengths of plastic tubing inserted in my chest to allow fluids to run out—I'll have to wear for several weeks. Glancing around the department store, I see mostly body-conscious, fitted styles. Without enough fabric to conceal the grenade-shaped bulbs collecting fluids, I'll look like a shoplifter from the military surplus store.

"What about this?" Mom holds up an ugly blouse—a boxy chambray camp-style with butterfly appliques—that might be the latest rage at the nursing home. I shake my head and make a gagging noise.

After much searching, we find a few baggy, short-sleeve shirts. They aren't exactly my favorites, but there's not much else available.

Next, we stop in Lingerie, where I find silky, jewel-toned pajamas, as well as some soft floral nightgowns.

After ringing up my purchases, Mom and I gravitate to Shoes, where all the sandals have been marked down.

Gotta love cute shoes. They always look good, even when you've gained a few pounds.

"Look at these." Mom holds up a pair of platform slides.

"Ooh, I love those!"

My mom is in her mid-60s, but you'd never guess it by looking at her or snooping in her closet. No old-lady shoes or stretchy pastel polyester pants for her. As a slender, striking teenager with wide eyes and delicate facial features, my mother was approached by a Hollywood agent who wanted her parents' permission for a screen test. But my conservative grandparents declined, not considering acting an appropriate profession for their daughter.

I tease Mom about this from time to time. Just think, instead of being a suburban homemaker, I could be a tacky Hollywood heiress with my own reality show. I'd spend my days getting hair extensions and spray-on tans, taunting the paparazzi. Sure, I might go club-hopping with my Eurotrash boyfriend, but at least I'd have enough class to remember to wear some La Perla panties under my Armani miniskirt when climbing out of limousines.

~

Several hours later, our arms loaded with packages, we head for the exit door in the Lingerie department. But then we spot another clearance sign. Tucked back in the corner are incredible markdowns. On one table there are bins of bikini briefs, hipsters, and boy shorts.

"How did we miss all this?" I ask.

"Look," Mom holds up a pair of silky underpants. "They have some really nice brands."

"What do you think of these?" I hold up a pair of enormous white granny-panties.

"I don't think so."

"Maybe you'd prefer this," I laugh, holding up a lacy purple thong.

Her face turns red. "Not my style either. Maybe something in between."

We rummage through the merchandise, searching for particular sizes and styles.

Divine Secret: Prepare for your recovery period.

Plan ahead to make your recovery easier. Make sure you have comfy clothes, ample medical supplies, and toiletries. Fill your pantry and fridge with your favorite drinks and snacks. Stock up on DVDs and books to help keep you entertained. Let people know how they can help. Give yourself permission to rest and focus on healing.

I move to the adjacent table and face a tub of bras, where the irony seizes me. The high of my shopping adventure deflates like a punctured balloon.

It doesn't matter if these bras are recommended by Oprah.

Or that they are marked 80% off.

Today is not my day for bra shopping.

~

The next day, Mom and I go to a store that specializes in post-mastectomy bras and swimsuits. I need to buy some soft and stretchy post-surgical camisoles, tank tops with little pockets sewn inside to hide drainage bulbs.

Upon entering the Boobtique, a couple of sales clerks rush to our side. They are both mature ladies with thick *New Yawker* accents.

"We're looking for some camisoles," Mom says. "And I think my daughter would like to see some of your products."

"Who's your surgeon, doll?" asks Silver-Haired Saleslady.

When I mention Rock Star Surgeon, they nod in approval.

"Oh, he's one of the best! A lot of our ladies have used him," says Red-Headed Saleslady.

"And I hear he's rather handsome," adds Silver-Haired Saleslady.

They lead me to a rack of camisoles, so I pick out two of the softest. Then they usher me past shelves stacked with prosthesis boxes. Displayed on the wall is an assortment of post-mastectomy bras. I cringe, because some look matronly, all huge and white with noticeable seams.

Silver-Haired Saleslady holds up one bra. "This is one of our best sellers."

It's beige with generous lace-trimmed cups that look like they would extend to my collar-bone.

"Thanks, but I'm used to a different style." I sigh. "Won't those seams show through t-shirts? I don't want to change my entire wardrobe."

"Oh, no, they'll work just fine." Red-Headed Saleslady points to her chest. "I'm wearing one right now and you can't tell. But we have seamless ones too. And different styles we can order."

"There's someone I want you to meet," says Silver-Haired Saleslady. She introduces me to their newest employee, a younger woman, maybe mid-30s, with long brunette hair.

"She's wearing a mastectomy bra and prosthesis!"

"Really?" I wouldn't have guessed.

Brunette Salesgirl has a medium-sized bustline. Her blouse is a silky geometric print with a scoop neckline. While it's not low-cut, it's not dowdy either.

"Hi," says Brunette Salesgirl. "I had some of the same concerns."

"Maybe you could show me your swimsuits and other products?" Mom asks the older salesladies. "Let's give these two a little time to talk."

Brunette Salesgirl and I compare notes.

"I had a single mastectomy three years ago," she confides. "But I haven't had any reconstruction done yet."

She explains that she's gotten used to wearing a prosthetic, that it hasn't been that bad. That the silicone breast form works with most of her clothes.

"And I was lucky, too," she says, "in that my hair grew back thick and fast after chemo." She opens a box and pulls out a breast form. "Go ahead, touch it."

I poke it with my index finger. It's somewhat jiggly, resembling a triangle.

"The forms come in different shapes and sizes to match your remaining breast," she says. "If you have a bilateral, then you can choose a pair of whatever size you want."

I look at her, open to encouragement. She reaches into a rack and pulls out satiny, seamless post-mastectomy bras.

"Our younger customers really like these," she says. "Trust me, once you're dressed, no one will know what's underneath just by looking."

"Thank you," I say. "You're definitely making me feel better."

"Good. I promise it won't be as bad as you fear."

"That's a relief. And I'm happy to see prettier bras, too."

"Glad to help. But in retrospect," she confesses, "I wish I'd had a bilateral. I found a lump in my remaining breast last week. I've got an appointment with my surgeon in a few days. Maybe it's just a cyst, but I can't stop worrying."

"I hope everything turns out okay." It sounds like she might be facing the scenario I fear, of having to go through the whole cancer crisis a second time. "Thanks again and good luck."

Mom and the two older salesladies return to the bra area. "Joanna, they've got some cute swimsuits in the other room."

I hedge—bathing suit shopping is the one retail excursion I dread.

"We have wigs upstairs too, if you'd like to try some on," adds Silver-Haired Saleslady.

Divine Secret: Search out stylish new options.

The Boobtique carried cream-of-the-crop merchandise, but several years ago, the pickings were slim. These days, you can find post-mastectomy bras in all sorts of designer colors.

"What do you think?" asks Mom.

"Sure. It might be fun."

Unfortunately, unlike the plethora of post-mastectomy bras, the wig selection at the Boobtique is rather paltry.

I tuck my hair under a hairnet, pull on a dark blonde wig, and look into the mirror.

Sha-zam! The layered shag style turns me into a 70s sitcom mom. I'm Florence Henderson of the Brady Bunch. *Here's the story, of a lovely lady...*

Next, I try on a light brunette bob with bangs. With a Versace pantsuit and oversize sunglasses, I could go trick-or-treating as Anna Wintour, legendary editor of *Vogue*.

Finally, I try on a layered golden blonde wig. It's closer to the color and style of my current hair but shorter.

"That's not bad," Mom says.

"But not exactly good."

I sigh. For once, I am sick and tired of shopping.

DS

Divine Secret: Seek out support.

For someone with cancer, I'm pretty damned lucky! I have good medical insurance, my husband's income covers our household expenses, and I have a network of friends and family willing to offer both practical and emotional support.

Not everyone has people lining up to help. Maybe you're new to an area, don't have any family nearby, or are the sole wage-earner for your household. Please understand, the amount of support you receive is not a popularity contest. It has more to do with how connected you are within a community.

I don't want to seem all Marie Antoinette-ish—cluelessly advising you to eat cake during a bread shortage—lacking compassion for those in different circumstances. I worry about my Pink Sisters overburdened with workplace and household responsibilities, who don't have a lot of resources. Who are single parents. Who don't have any family living nearby. Who have to drag themselves to their jobs on days they're depleted from chemo. Who have to deal with laundry, housework, etc. while recovering from surgery.

And I worry about my Pink Sisters who don't have insurance or can't afford to pay for prescriptions and treatments. Every single person on the globe, no matter how competent or powerful, will face moments of vulnerability—times when it seems impossible to go it alone.

Pink Sisters, the world is not always a cruel and cold place. It's okay to ask for help. Do it pro-actively; don't wait until you are struggling and feeling isolated. Take a leap of faith and contact possible resources:

* Nurse navigators and hospital social workers
* Local churches, many of which operate casserole ministries
* A few loud-mouthed but big-hearted neighbors—you'll be surprised how people will rally
* Local cancer support groups

Also, employee assistance programs may offer donated sick leave contributions. Remember, someday you'll get the chance to pay it forward, to help another Pink Sister in need, so don't let pride or shyness stop you from asking for a helping hand.

I'd Like to Phone a Friend

Okay, I've told most of my closest friends and neighbors. There are a few more calls I have to make, but I keep procrastinating. I need to tell Beth and Mary Lou, my dear friends in Texas.

Beth and I met when we were both new mothers. I was drawn to her warm and witty sense of humor. With a natural charm, Beth can start a conversation with a stranger, and before you know it, they're laughing like old friends. In fact, her first job after college was in adult beverage marketing, which meant she was paid to chat up guys in bars and get them to try her company's beer.

Beth and I have always had an easy, yet deep, connection. We can talk about anything and usually understand each other's viewpoint. She took care of Alex when I went to the hospital to have Nick. Even though our family has moved away from Texas, I try to see Beth and her daughter as often as possible. We've spent time together on vacation with our kids as well as on mom-only trips.

It's hard to tell Beth about my cancer because she'll care so much. I mean, I'm lucky to have many friends and neighbors who're worried about me. But if something bad happens, Beth would really, really miss me. Also, I hate to give her more unhappy news. She's recently divorced. Her dad has been seriously ill for months and her oldest brother is battling kidney cancer.

I finally summon the nerve and call her.

"Hey, Beth."

"Hi there! What have the Chapmans been up to?"

"All kinds of stuff."

I ask about her dad. Her brother. Her daughter. Her new job. If she's met any cute single guys.

"No, no time or energy for that," she replies. "But are you ready to plan our next vacation? I'm thinking white sandy beaches and clear turquoise water."

"Sounds perfect! I'll definitely need a fun trip before long."

"Jo, what's going on?" Her tone turns serious. She hears the strain in my voice.

I hesitate for a second.

"I have breast cancer. Luckily, the doctors believe it was caught early. So I should have an excellent prognosis. But I have to have surgery—a mastectomy—soon. Then possibly chemo."

"No!" she cries. "Don't you tell me that! No, that is simply not acceptable."

"I know."

"I can't deal with any more sick people in my life," she wails. "Don't you know I've reached my quota?"

"Sorry to inconvenience you," I laugh.

"Yeah, some friend you are," she jokes.

"I've been meaning to call you," I confess. "I've been putting it off because I dreaded telling you."

"It's about time you did! I really can't believe this. You know I'm coming out to see you."

"That would be great. My mom will be here during and after surgery. Maybe you could fly out here and cheer me up after a chemo session."

"You can count on it. I'll even hold your barf bag."

"Now that's the sign of a true friend."

"We *are* true friends! Jo, seriously, I'm so sorry this is going on. What else can I do?"

"Ask your dad to put me on his prayer list." Beth's dad is a retired Presbyterian minister. "I figure he's got the hotline."

"Don't worry, you'll get bumped to the top!"

I fill in the gory details. After we hang up, I close my eyes for an instant, grateful for a friend like Beth.

~

I need a break, so I walk downstairs to get a cup of tea.

"One call down, one to go," I tell Ryan.

A few moments later, I'm holding the phone, preparing to call Mary Lou. We were college roommates who turned into life-long friends. Over the past thirty years, we've been there for each other through lousy boyfriends, good husbands, family troubles, and child-rearing challenges.

We actually won the "messiest room" award in our sorority house, which we proudly displayed on Parents Weekend. I remember when Mary Lou developed a huge crush on Joe, the graduate student teaching her 8 a.m. martial arts class. Normally, Mary Lou would sleep in until the last minute, then race to class. But for Joe's classes, she'd wake up early, making time to put her hair in hot rollers and apply makeup.

Sometimes we'd try to think up martial arts questions so she'd have an excuse to call Joe. I can't remember the questions now, but I imagine they were pretty lame. He kept a respectful distance until the semester was over, then fell in love with her.

Honestly, who wouldn't? Mary Lou has an uncanny knack for finding the silver lining in the darkest cloud. Her sunny disposition and enthusiasm are infectious; my mood is always elevated when I'm around her.

We are Aunt Jo and Uncle Ryan to Mary Lou's kids, connected by heartstrings, not bloodlines.

However, despite her unwavering optimism, Mary Lou has been dealing with challenging health issues within her own family. I hate to add more bad news to her life. But finally, I dial her number.

"Hey, girlfriend," she says. "How's everything?"

"Busy as usual." I ask about her three children, her husband, and her parents. I give her updates on Alex, Nick, and Larissa. Then I drop the bombshell. "I have something to tell you. I've been diagnosed with breast cancer."

"What? Are you kidding me?"

"No, I'm afraid not."

"Oh, Joanna," she sobs. "Oh, no!"

My heart twists like a wrung-out washcloth. I can hear the sounds of her crying.

"No! No!"

"It's going to be okay," I reassure her. "The doctors believe they've caught it early. I should be fine."

"I'm so sorry. And so worried! How are Ryan and the kids taking this?"

"Kids are a little nervous but seem okay. You know Ryan lost his mom to cancer, so this stirs up bad memories."

"I can't believe this," she says, her words coming out snuffled. "What can I do?"

"Just having you as a friend is a huge help."

"I would do anything for you. Just anything."

"You'll take my delightful children if I kick the bucket and Ryan gets run over by a bus?"

"Don't say that!"

"Just kidding," I say. "We're going to be great-grandmas together someday. We'll do chair yoga and play Bingo."

"Yes, we'll rock the nursing home!" she sniffles. "And you know I'd take your kids in a heartbeat."

"I know and I love you for it. I'd take yours, too."

"I love you, too. I can't believe this is happening!"

I can hear her crying, and it shreds my insides. "I'm going to be fine."

I keep reassuring her until she calms down. I have friends who'd miss me, but my death would leave a gaping hole in her heart, just like hers would in mine.

After we hang up, I go in the bedroom and sprawl on the bed, emotionally spent. Ryan walks in a few minutes later.

"Did you reach Mary Lou?"

"I did. It was hard, though. She couldn't stop crying."

"She's worried." He lies down on the bed beside me. "I know it was tough, but they need to know."

There are more people I should probably call, because they'd want to know: my college friend living in Colorado, my roommate from grad school, my neighbor who moved to Florida, my writing group back in Texas. But I'm emotionally drained. I don't want to talk any more.

~

We host Nick's birthday party at the YMCA a week early since I'll be in the hospital on his actual birthday. We've rented a bounce house, plus the boys get to play basketball. His friends are sports nuts, kids from our neighborhood as well as former YMCA basketball teammates. Brandon, a close friend of Nick's who recently moved out of the state, is back in town for a visit. He's been staying with us some while his parents are on vacation.

Walking from the gym to the party room, I greet Dr. Point Guard when he drops off his son for Nick's party.

"Are you doing okay?"

"Yeah, I'm in countdown mode," I reply. "But when I talked to my surgeon, he wasn't keen on installing a port." I shake my head, hoping my doctors don't end up in a pissing contest.

Dr. Point Guard grabs my wrists and turns them so the undersides of my forearms are exposed.

"Hmm," he says, tapping my wrist. "Your veins look pretty good."

Okay, it's a little weird that he's examining my veins at Nick's birthday party.

He explains he'd likely prescribe a chemo regimen requiring only four infusion sessions—none of them with Adriamyacin, often nicknamed the "red devil"—a harsh chemical caustic to skin.

"You'd do fine with an IV," he continues. "But if you need a port, we can do it at our facility. It would be an easy outpatient procedure."

He suggests I could use Kathleen's husband, Dr. Gravitas, a lanky radiologist, to insert the port, not noticing my wince. I've already broken my rule of not using doctors I know socially. Not sure I want every friend in the medical profession seeing me unconscious, splayed out like a side of beef.

~

The next night, I'm in the bathroom applying makeup when Ryan comes in. Brandon's parents are in town to pick him up and are flying back home the following day. Their former neighbors are hosting a cocktail party, and we've been invited.

"Hey," he asks, leaning in the doorway. "How badly do you want to go to the party tonight?"

"I've been looking forward to seeing Lynette and Doug. It should be fun."

He sighs. I halt my mascara wand mid-air.

"Honey, I'm sorry, but I just don't want to go."

I put down the mascara and turn toward him. His blue eyes look tired and sad.

"I know you want to see them," he continues. "I like them, too. But I don't feel like socializing. You're having surgery soon. I don't have the energy to act happy and talk to people."

Divine Secret: Remember that it's emotionally exhausting for your loved ones, too.

You're not the only one stressed and scared. Try to take into account the feelings of your spouse, friends, caretakers, etc. Everyone is focused on you and your feelings, but they're having a hard time, too, and may not feel comfortable sharing their anxieties.

"Okay," I say. "I understand. Let's stay home."

That night we sit close together on the couch holding hands, watching a forgettable movie on the DVD player. I'd been so wrapped up in my own emotions and in keeping tabs on the kids that I'd underestimated how hard this was for my husband. But tonight we're together and that's all that matters.

Resource: Book

Breast Cancer Husband: How to Help Your Wife (And Yourself) during Diagnosis, Treatment and Beyond, by Marc Silver

Whose Number Is That On My Caller ID?

August 2007

Approximately five weeks after my diagnosis, it's time for my pre-surgical appointment. I'm glad I stuck with an oncology surgeon, but the long wait has rattled me. I'm beyond ready to have the cancer removed.

It's still scary to sit in a waiting room at the cancer center. I can't help but wonder about the people around me. *What type of cancer do they have? Is their prognosis better or worse than mine?*

Before long, Caring Nurse escorts me to an exam room. Rock Star Surgeon goes over the procedure and outlines a recovery timeline for the mastectomy as well as the sentinel node biopsy.

"I'll be doing a skin-sparing operation," he explains, warning me that the remaining folds of skin may look strange—not like photos of survivors with taut, scarred chests—but allow for a better appearance after reconstruction.

Who knows how long that will be? I don't want to think about it anymore.

He reminds me to limit activity and refrain from lifting during my recovery. He mentions the drains that will need to stay in my chest until the amount of fluid decreases. I've only ever spent a few nights in the hospital—when I gave birth to my sons—so I can't help feeling a little anxious. "I'm still worried about the second tumor."

"I don't think it will change anything. Both tumors look small."

He asks me if I have questions, but I think I know what to expect.

Leaving the surgeon's office, I cross the street for pre-surgical tests at the hospital. After filling out a sheaf of paperwork, I wait in another lobby until called.

A nurse anesthetist questions me about prior experience with anesthesia, existing medical problems, possible allergies to latex, and current medications.

"Do not eat or drink anything after midnight on the evening before surgery," she warns me. "This is critical! Nothing to eat or drink after midnight."

"Okay." Guess we won't be stopping off at Waffle House on the way to the hospital.

A different nurse enters the room. "Hi, I'm going to do an EKG to check your heart," she explains. I unbutton my shirt and recline on the exam table. Round sensors stuck like band-aids to my body record my heart rhythm. Yet another test I've never had before.

Next, I'm escorted down the hallway, where a phlebotomist draws several vials of blood. I'm instructed to follow the signs on a maze-like path to Radiology, where I get chest X-rays. Finally, I'm done.

Only a few days left until surgery, so I help Alex and Nick pack for the cruise. I buy back-to-school supplies and catch up on laundry. I double up recipes, storing casseroles in the freezer.

~

Two nights before my mastectomy, the phone rings at 7 p.m. I pick up the receiver, surprised to hear Rock Star Surgeon on the line.

"Hi, how are you?" I ask, on cheery default mode.

"Fine," he answers. "But I'm afraid I'm not calling to chat."

Duh, how slow on the uptake am I? Surgeons don't call to shoot the breeze!

Rock Star Surgeon's voice sounds somber.

"Oh." I feel jittery, like I've chugged a thermos of coffee.

"I hate to tell you this, but there's a suspicious spot on one of your lungs."

"Oh, no." I'm spinning, falling, out of control. Powerless to stop this terrifying descent, like I've been pushed off the edge of the Grand Canyon.

"Many times something like this turns out benign, but we need to investigate before I can perform your surgery."

"You think it's lung cancer? Will you do another biopsy?"

"It's more likely to be metastatic breast cancer than a primary lung cancer, meaning that the cancer from the breast has spread to your lung. We don't know anything for sure. The first step is to get a CT scan. I'll schedule you in STAT, wherever we can get you in the quickest. I'll call you with results as soon as I know something."

"Okay, thanks."

Why am I thanking him? Strange to say this automatically, after being told I might have Stage IV cancer.

"I'm sorry," Rock Star Surgeon says. "I hated making this call to you, but I don't deal the cards. All I can do is play the hand dealt."

Well then, I hope he's a ferocious card shark, like one of those brainy MIT students who beat the Vegas dealers in blackjack.

Hanging up the phone, I have a weird feeling of detachment, like one of those out-of-body experiences, where I'm watching from an outsider's perspective. I realize Rock Star Surgeon might not operate if I have metastatic disease. Current medical thinking is mastectomy after the cancer has infiltrated other organs is like locking the barn after the horse has already escaped.

I lean over the top of the staircase. "Ryan, come here! I have to tell you something."

He bolts upstairs. I close our bedroom door.

"What's going on?" Unnerved by my insistence and strange expression, he looks worried.

"The phone call…they saw something in my lungs. It might be Stage IV cancer. I have to have a CT scan tomorrow."

"You're kidding." His expression looks frozen as he tries to comprehend what I'm saying. "No, no," he shakes his head and his face crumples.

"This can't be happening," I say.

Ryan wraps his arms around me. "We don't know anything for sure yet."

Starting to panic, I pull away, telling him I need to call Dr. Point Guard. Most physicians don't give out their pager numbers to patients—it's sort of like the Bat Phone—so I'm glad to have the inside track. I leave a frantic message, hoping he'll call back soon.

The shock transforms into visceral fear, clawing my innards. *Has cancer invaded my vital organs, digging in deep, holding on with an iron-clad grasp?*

I try to calm myself. From conversations with my *YSC* Sisters, I know some Stage IV survivors live for many years with a decent quality of life. *But is this the exception, not the rule?*

New drugs may halt progression or even bring about a health status called NED, No Evidence of Disease. As a Stage IV survivor, you can't give up hope, but the odds are not in your favor. Once cancer has metastasized, it's likely to be the cause of your death. Newer drugs might buy months or years of survival, but probably not decades.

If the cancer's spread to my lungs, it could be slowed, but not eradicated. I shiver with a cold chill, and sharp pains pierce my stomach, as if vultures were feasting on my organs, leaving behind only bone.

How is it that death may have crept in so quietly, like a stealthy cat-burglar?

The thought of not being here for my kids devastates me. If I'm Stage IV, I'll hang on to hope, but there are limits to modern medicine. New drug trials happen each day, but it's a race against the clock. Hoping, hoping, hoping for a cure.

Tears and panic overwhelm me like a tidal wave I cannot stop. Every day, children around the world lose their mothers to violence, famine, or disease. It's not fair and sometimes shakes my faith in God. And cancer is cruel, random. *Will Anyone answer my prayer? Or is my plea rolling over to celestial voicemail?*

If I were God, I'd be annoyed by humans who ignore Me most of the time, then plead for divine intervention when tragedy strikes. Maybe we believe too much in self-determination, that we can carve out our own destiny. Yet all it takes is one missed stop sign, a rickety ladder, or a nasty virus to irrevocably damage—or end—your life or the lives of those you love. We blithely live as if there's a steel-reinforced, concrete barrier protecting us from mortality, but it's just a flimsy plastic shower curtain that can be ripped down at any second.

I know we all die sometime, but I have my future mapped out. I want to cheer at graduations, dance at weddings, hold my newborn grandchildren. I want to grow older and crankier with Ryan. To someday go to the early-bird dinners and join a square-dance club. I want to prepare holiday feasts for my grandkids, complete with my traditional Cajun-blackened (aka burnt) rolls.

Within minutes, Surgery Scheduler calls me with a location for the CT scan, scheduled for 7 a.m. tomorrow. Mom is planning to arrive in the afternoon, but I'll need her in the morning.

I pick up the phone, trying to keep my voice calm. "Hi, Mom. Any way you could get here earlier?"

"I've got a few errands. I was thinking around one or two."

"Can you make it earlier?"

"Maybe around eleven?"

I have to tell her. "Please don't worry, but I need you here early. During my pre-op screening, they saw a suspicious spot on my lung. I have to have a chest CT at 7 a.m. Then maybe a biopsy."

"They think you have lung cancer?"

"No. It's more likely to be metastatic breast cancer."

I know she's grappling to understand. This is one of the most confusing aspects of the disease. Tumors can spread to lungs, liver, brain, or bones, but it's still breast cancer, regardless of the site. At that point the cancer is Stage IV. There is no Stage V.

"Oh, no," she replies. "I'll start packing now. I'm coming tonight."

~

Dr. Point Guard hasn't called back, so I phone Kathleen's husband, Dr. Gravitas, asking for help in tracking him down. Dr. Gravitas is a nice man, albeit with a serious demeanor. No one would mistake him for Robin Williams with a clown nose.

Dr. Gravitas explains that Dr. Point Guard is on a family vacation and probably silenced his pager.

"Sorry to bother you at home, but I just got some scary news."

"What's wrong?"

"I-I-I," choking on the words, I can barely breathe. Overcome by sobs, I cannot speak.

"Joanna? Joanna? Are you okay?"

"It-it-it might be Stage IV," I sputter. "They saw something on my lung. I have to get a CT scan."

"Are you getting it done here?"

The downtown medical center where Rock Star Surgeon operates has recently acquired several smaller hospitals, including the one where Dr. Point Guard and Dr. Gravitas practice. However, despite the merger, there are still kinks in sharing information electronically.

"No, they scheduled me at another branch, wherever they could find the earliest available slot."

"When you go in," Dr. Gravitas instructs me, "take a CD and ask for a copy of the scan, then call me. I'll meet you at my office and tell you what I see."

"Thank you," I cry. "Really, thank you so much!"

I'm very grateful to him. Otherwise, I'd be in a terrifying

limbo, possibly waiting hours for a random radiologist to read my scan, make the report, and share the results with Rock Star Surgeon. No telling how long before I'd hear something. If there's terrible news, I'd rather hear it from Dr. Gravitas than a stranger.

~

Ten minutes later, Dr. Point Guard calls. "I'm sorry, but I had my pager turned off briefly. I don't do that very often."

"That's okay. I'm sorry to bother you on vacation."

"No, no," he insists. "My patients are like family. Tell me what's going on."

"My surgeon called. He sees a spot on my lung. Thinks it could be metastatic cancer." I tell him about my impending CT scan and Dr. Gravitas's offer to immediately review my results.

> **Divine Secret: Use those personal connections.**
>
> I've changed my tune about mixing personal and professional aspects of life. It's nice to be treated by physicians who know you as an individual, especially when facing a serious health crisis. If you have personal connections, use them! It's good to be a VIP, even if it's in the cancer ward.

Dr. Point Guard listens empathetically, reminding me we don't know anything for certain. It could be a false alarm, an anomaly with no clinical significance.

"I'll call you early tomorrow morning," he says. "I've got my laptop with me, so I can look at the scans once you get them to our radiology department. I know it's hard, but try not to worry too much. We're going to hope and pray that whatever they're seeing in your lung is benign."

It Could Be Worse

What if I don't survive?

All night, I toss and turn, squinting at the illuminated numbers on my bedside clock. I ask God's forgiveness for my sins: when I've harbored a grudge, made snarky comments, or yelled at my kids. I promise to be a better mom, better wife, better friend, better Christian. I'll give more money to church. Be more patient with my family and less judgmental of others. I'll even start returning library books on time. *Can't we reach some sort of bargain?*

~

It's still dark outside as we prepare to leave for the CT scan. Ryan pours a cup of coffee but I'm already too rattled to tolerate caffeine. I give Mom a quick hug on our way out the door.

On the ride to the designated medical center, Ryan and I are mostly silent, except for my grim predictions. One of my coping mechanisms has always been to prepare for the worst-case scenario, but this strategy is not helping me now.

"I bet I'm Stage IV. I bet it's in my lungs."

"Don't say that!" Ryan pleads. "We don't know."

I sway back and forth in my seat like a distraught child.

~

The sun is rising as we enter the hospital. At the admissions desk, the clerk seems confused and can't locate our paperwork. I keep telling her my CT scan was scheduled last night, ordered STAT. Finally, she calls Radiology and they tell her to send me back.

A nurse meets me at the door. She gives me a Styrofoam cup filled with a vile beverage of barium contrast suspension. "You need to drink this before the test."

I take a swallow. *Yuck!* The fruit flavoring can't mask the metallic taste or the chalky texture. I start to dry heave.

"Take a deep breath," the nurse says. "I'm sorry, but you have to drink it all. Do you want to take it to the waiting room? Maybe watch a little TV to distract yourself while you're drinking it?"

"Yes. Thank you."

Walking back to the lobby, I see a number of people holding the tell-tale cup.

I slump in the chair next to Ryan. He raises his eyebrows, surprised at my quick return.

"I have to drink this nasty stuff first. I gagged at the first sip." Maybe if the stakes weren't so high, it'd be easier to choke it down, but the test might reveal cancer's tentacles unfurling throughout my body.

"Just take it easy," he urges me. "A little bit at a time."

On the overhead television, news commentators yammer. My brain is in a state of disequilibrium, and I cannot understand anything they're saying. A desperate mantra—please be okay, please be okay, please be okay—echoes through my mind.

I concentrate on calming my roiling stomach and forcing down the drink. When the cup is nearly empty, I notify the nurse.

"Come on back," she says, buzzing me in.

"Can my husband come, too?"

"He can't be in the room during the scan, but he can wait in the hallway."

Ryan and I walk down the corridor to where the CT machine is housed.

The radiology technician comes out from the control room to introduce himself. Ryan hands him the blank CD.

"Would you make a copy of my wife's results?"

"Well, I guess I can," he replies, his tone uncertain.

Moments later, I'm reclined on an exam table while the CT scanner, a horseshoe-like structure, records multiple views of my organs.

As the machine hums and thumps, I'm in a state of disbelief. *How could my positive prognosis turn grim so quickly?* I'm not ready to say goodbye to my children, my family, my friends.

In a matter of minutes the test is done.

Now I have to wait for results, the key to my future. *Are the malignant cells confined to my breast? Or have they crept into other organs? At this point, can doctors still eradicate the cancer from my body? Or, at best, slow down the spread?*

As trained, the technician maintains a poker face, disclosing nothing.

"The copy, please?" Ryan reminds him.

He hands us the disc and we leave.

We hurry to the parking lot while Ryan dials Dr. Gravitas's cell. He picks up immediately.

"We've got a copy of the scans."

"Good. I'll meet you there."

Ryan accelerates out of the parking lot. We're both on edge, our hearts racing. I look at the commuters yawning in nearby cars, on their way to another routine workday. Probably none of them are driving somewhere to learn their fate, their chance for survival.

I want to be hopeful, but I need to prepare for bad news. If I have to, I'll look for a back-up plan, maybe a clinical trial somewhere.

Please, God, don't let this be Stage IV. Don't let it have spread to my lungs!

Midway through the drive, my cell phone rings, startling me.

I don't recognize the number, but answer it anyway. It's Rock Star Surgeon.

"Good news," he says. "Report says it appears to be a granulated nodule, no evidence of metastatic cancer. Probably the result of a previous respiratory infection."

"Really? That's great!"

"Yes, I was very happy to hear. Don't worry anymore. I'll see you early tomorrow morning."

"Thank you!"

I turn to Ryan and smile. "Everything looks fine. No cancer in my lungs."

Exhaling loudly, he touches the roof. "Thank God!" He leans across the console and gives me a quick kiss. "Best news ever."

I call Mom. "Everything's okay. Still on for surgery tomorrow."

"Oh, what a relief! I was so worried."

"Me, too."

I call Dr. Gravitas and Dr. Point Guard to tell them my happy results.

Thank God, the cancer is ONLY in my breast!

Divine Secret: Your definition of good news may change.

In a perfect world, no one would receive a cancer diagnosis. But we know the world is far from perfect. To an outsider, sometimes the good news may seem a small victory, far less than remission or healing. Perhaps you're in a place where you're grateful for a slowed progression, better tolerance of treatments, or a stabilized health situation. Still, you and your Pink Sisters rejoice.

A Letter to My Sisters with Metastatic (Stage IV) Cancer

My dear Sisters,

I don't know what to say.

There are no words to make it better.

I'm afraid anything I say will sound trite, obtuse, or insensitive.

But I want you to know that I'm thinking of you and wishing I could make it better.

Admittedly, I'm profoundly relieved to learn the suspicious spot on my lung is not metastatic breast cancer. Yet, I feel a bittersweet twinge, because for some of you, the test results will not be reassuring. You may be advised to endure more scans, more surgeries, and more drug treatments to slow the cancer's progression and prolong your life.

People in pink shirts run for the cure, walk for the cure, participate in clinical trials, donate money to research foundations. And progress is being made. Almost every day, medical journals buzz with data on newer drugs and promising clinical trials. Some scientists are even trying to develop a breast cancer vaccine. I have to believe that, someday soon, there will be a cure.

But the cure may not come soon enough for you. There's not an appropriate Hallmark card for this occasion. A "get well soon" card sounds stupid or insensitive.

I had the hardest time knowing what to say to Christine, the beautiful and brave mom who died less than two years after traveling with us to China. Their family thought she'd beaten her rare and aggressive cancer, but it roared back with a vengeance to claim her life.

After our Myrtle Beach reunion, Jeff, Christine, and their girls had an extremely early flight home. The night before, they'd gone to everyone's room to say goodbye, but I'd been in the shower. I couldn't sleep, so around 5 a.m., I got up and went to the lobby. I poured a cup of coffee and pretended to read the newspaper while staking out the reception desk.

When Christine and her family checked out, I walked over to say goodbye. I can still remember the intensity of that hug. I knew somehow it would be the last time I'd see her.

Over the next few months, as her health deteriorated, I called a few times, but stumbled over what to say, what to ask. Every time I mailed Christine a card, I struggled over what to write. In my last message I told her I hoped she had a beautiful view from her bedroom window and that her pain was under control.

It's not much, but it was the best I could do.

Maybe this is lame, but here's what I wish for you, my Stage IV Sisters: that you don't lose hope and can maintain a good quality of life. Always remember that you are not a statistic. May you be one of the survivors who outlives all expectations.

Life can be lonely and sad when you have metastatic disease, when people don't know what to say or do to comfort you, when they back away as if your condition is contagious.

I wish I could wrap you up in a fuzzy knit blanket of your favorite color—which I'm guessing is probably not pink. I'd sit you down beside a cozy fire and bring you hot chai tea and chocolate croissants. Fill your bookshelves with new releases from your favorite authors and your iPod with soothing music. Invite your closest friends over—the ones who could make you laugh, but would also let you curse and cry.

When you were tired, I'd help you to a comfy bedroom overlooking the ocean, where the sounds of the waves could lull you to sleep. I'd scatter scented candles and framed photos of your favorite memories on the dresser and nightstand. I'd help you write letters to your loved ones. I'd hold your hand whenever you were scared, until you no longer needed me.

Thinking of you, wishing you fortitude, comfort, and peace.

Love,
Joanna

My Own Personal D-Day

The alarm rings at 4:30 a.m; it's completely dark outside. I've had a fitful night of sleep, grim dreams constantly intruding. Solemn, sad, and determined, I shower with the special antibacterial soap they'd instructed me to use. I rub the lather across my chest, realizing my body will soon undergo irrevocable change.

Drying off, I look into the mirror. It's hard to comprehend that my breast, free of pain and appearing normal, except for a small biopsy scar, harbors a lethal disease. Again, I pray the malignant cells are contained within my breast and haven't spread.

I dress in yoga pants and a baggy zip-up sweater; I let my bra fall to the floor of the closet. I won't need it anytime soon.

The kids are asleep, so we keep our voices low. Ryan pours himself a cup of coffee, but I'm not allowed to eat or drink anything. Mom waits downstairs in her robe.

"Joanna, I'm sure everything will go fine," she says. "I'll be there as soon as I get the kids off to school."

She's putting on a brave face, but her eyes look tired and worried.

"Pop already left. He'll be at the hospital in a few hours," she adds. "Ryan, call me with updates."

I give her a big hug before walking out the door.

The houses on our street are dark. No one's awake except shift workers and insomniacs. We drive in silence. I don't think either one of us knows what to say. The cloak of pre-dawn darkness, the anxious anticipation, the willful summoning of grit give me a strange feeling of affinity to those young and terrified soldiers in the moments before storming the beaches of Normandy.

I look out the windows at the lighted skyscrapers. When the silence becomes unbearable, Ryan turns on the radio. The DJs banter, but they could be speaking in Farsi for all I hear. Finally, we pull into the hospital parking lot.

"How about I bring your suitcase in later?"

"That's fine." After all, I'll be wearing a lovely wraparound hospital gown for the immediate future.

Only a handful of cars are parked in the patient garage. At the surgical reception desk, a clerk fastens a plastic ID bracelet around my wrist and hands me a pager.

I sit beside Ryan in the lobby. As usual, I've brought plenty of reading material: *Redbook*, *Time*, and a book, *40 Ways to Look at Winston Churchill: A Brief Account of a Long Life*. I flip aimlessly through the magazines, unable to focus on any of the articles or accompanying photographs.

When reading fails me, I start playing the "it could be worse" mind-game, my idiosyncratic and dysfunctional method of coping with unpleasant situations. What if I lived in a strict Islamic country, my body cloaked in a burka, forbidden to undress before a male doctor? What if I lived in a poor African village, with no running water, electricity, or medical personnel? I should be *grateful* that I'm being treated by skilled physicians in a modern medical facility, my expenses covered by health insurance. My chances of survival are enormously better than in many places on this earth. Perhaps this is just a bump in the road. Maybe I'll live a long and healthy life.

I put the magazines aside and pick up the Churchill biography. I've always been fascinated by the battlefields and home fronts during WWII. Somehow, the citizens of Great Britain soldiered through each terrible day. At night, they'd pull the blackout shades and huddle in subway stations as the air sirens screamed. *Keep calm and carry on.* Indeed.

I need that stiff upper lip to do what must be done. Yes, I'm losing a breast, but at least I'm not sending my sons to war or watching bombs destroy my family home.

After a short wait, the pager goes off. A nurse meets us at the door to the pre-operative area.

"Sir, you'll need to remain in the waiting room for now. It won't be long."

The pre-surgical area consists of a dozen curtained cubicles, each with a gurney and guest chair. Mine is directly across from the nurses' desk, where I can see the clock and multiple whiteboards.

The nurse points at a folded hospital gown. "Go ahead and change. Gown open in the front," she instructs. "I'll be back soon."

The curtain rings make a scraping sound as she pulls the drapes shut. Then, I'm alone in my cubicle. My nerves feel prickly, amped with adrenaline.

I remind myself that Hannah's husband works here, so when the nurse returns, I do a little name-dropping.

"You work with Will, right? The nurse anesthetist?" I ask. "He's a friend of mine."

"Oh, yes," she answers. "Nice guy. Great at his job."

"He promised you'd take good care of me."

"Of course we will!" She smiles and glances at her clipboard. "I need to ask a few questions. What's your name and birthdate?"

Easy enough. Still, she reads my ID bracelet for verification.

"Anything to eat or drink after midnight?"

"No."

"Any allergies to latex or rubber?"

"No."

She checks my vitals with a thermometer and blood pressure cuff, then rolls a small cart to my bedside.

"I'm going to go ahead and start the IV. Get some fluids in you. You'll also receive an antibiotic to help ward off infection."

I hate the snap of the thick rubber strap, the slaps to my forearm, wrist, and hand, the plunge of the needle. I turn my head until the nurse tells me it's done.

"Can I have my happy cocktail now?" I ask, thinking I could really use an intravenous elixir to bring down my anxiety.

"Not yet," she croons, as if I'm a child asking for cookies before dinner. "Your surgeon needs to talk to you first, but I'll get your husband."

Moments later, Ryan slips inside the cubicle. He's jittery and anxious, too, repeatedly checking the zipper of his laptop case before he sits down. He reaches for my hand. We look at each other, but the words aren't there.

The curtain parts, and Rock Star Surgeon strides in.

"Well, hello." After shaking my hand, then Ryan's, he points to a section of highlighted text on his clipboard. "Take a look."

It's the radiology report from my lung CT.

"I told you already, but I wanted you to see the official report. *Benign granular nodule.* Your lungs are good."

"We were so relieved. That was a scary moment."

"Me, too," he says, shaking his head. "I hate making those unwelcome phone calls. Was happy to have good news for you."

Flipping the page, he shows me a circular image representing the quadrants of my breast. He points out two marks that indicate the location of each tumor. "Today, I'll be performing a mastectomy of your right breast."

I nod. This statement must be standard operating procedure. Okay by me, because I don't want to wake up missing a leg or kidney.

Rock Star Surgeon gets a marker and starts drawing lines on my chest.

"Are you writing 'Take This One Off'?"

He looks at me strangely, not sure whether to laugh. Maybe he's thinking too much mirth might be inappropriate. I'm pretty certain he's decided I'm kind of wacky.

"I'll see you soon." Giving my shoulder a reassuring pat, he exits the cubicle.

I peek out the curtain and gesture for my nurse. "It's five o'clock somewhere! Time for my happy cocktail?"

"Just a little longer."

Next, I'm wheeled down the hall to the radiology area. I'm annoyed by this, because I am perfectly capable of walking there myself.

The sentinel node removal is a relatively new procedure. In years past, surgeons removed many lymph nodes, which could lead to lymphedema, a painful chronic swelling of the arm. Instead of performing the axillary node dissection, Rock Star Surgeon will remove only the nodes where cancer would spread first. If they are deemed cancer-free, no more nodes are taken.

Rolling into the treatment area, I'm pleasantly surprised to see Reluctant Radiologist, the doctor who interpreted my breast MRI results.

"Hi," I chirp. "Nice to see you again!"

Reluctant Radiologist looks startled, unaccustomed to patients greeting him as cheerfully as acquaintances re-connecting at a wedding reception or cocktail party.

"Remember me? I pestered you about my MRI."

"Yes, I do," he replies, his expression warming. "I'm glad our paths crossed again. I don't usually see patients multiple times." He explains that radiologists in his practice rotate between performing biopsies, reading scans, and assisting with surgical procedures.

"Thanks again for your help. I know I badgered you into talking, but I needed your opinion."

"Glad I could help," he says. "And today I'm trying something to relieve discomfort caused by the dye injections. I've been doing a trial using a local anesthetizing cream."

"Sounds good to me." I hate when doctors say something may cause discomfort. *Just call a spade a spade. Admit it will hurt!*

A nurse drapes me with a paper bib, then Reluctant Radiologist applies cream around my right nipple. After waiting a few minutes for the numbing to take effect, he holds up a syringe filled with blue radioactive dye and plunges it into the upper part of my areola. I feel a slight pinch and some pressure.

"How did that feel?"

"Not too bad, actually."

He injects the dye several more times in a clockwise fashion. "The dye will spread into your lymphatic system. During surgery, the doctors use radioactive tracers to find the sentinel nodes."

Sounds pretty cool, though I'm not thrilled about being radioactive.

"Still okay?"

"Hurting a little," I wince. "But not too bad."

He injects the dye one last time.

"Ow! Ow!"

I'm surprised by the sound of my voice crying out, gasping with pain. It feels like I've been stung in the nipple by a gigantic, mad-as-hell, sadistic queen bee.

"Sorry," he says. "Before I started using the anesthetizing cream, patients told me the sentinel node injections were the worst part of their surgical experience."

"Well, it definitely helped for the first few."

"Good. A bilateral requires eight injections, so in the past, I almost had to peel some of them off the ceiling."

"I'm glad they didn't all feel like that last one. Thanks again for your help."

"Good luck to you," Reluctant Radiologist replies, as the nurse pushes me back to the pre-surgical bay.

～

Ryan and I sit in the cubicle watching the clock. Surgery can't begin until the blue dye has moved to my lymph nodes.

The nurse pokes her head inside the curtain. "Your pastor is here. Do you want to see him?"

"Sure."

"They got you back here fast," Barry says, entering my partition. "I thought you'd still be in the waiting room."

Maybe to him it seems like an accelerated process, but to me each moment has been painfully long. I look at his laminated nametag. "You've got the backstage pass, huh?"

"Yeah," he laughs. "The people at the desk know me. But this is a great hospital. You're in good hands."

I'm glad he's here, but a little unnerved. *Aren't pastoral visits for seriously ill people?* His presence underscores the gravity of the situation.

We chat awhile about our kids, church, and mutual friends.

"How about a prayer?" Barry asks, reaching for my hand.

I reach for Ryan with my other hand. We form a small circle as Barry prays for healing and comfort, his words a balm to my spirit.

"Ryan, I'll be in the waiting room." He exits my curtained area with a handshake and a hug.

I'm glad Barry is staying with Ryan while I'm in surgery. Pop should be here soon.

～

We wait and wait and wait in my cubicle. I hear the rattle of other patients being wheeled to the operating room. I think about brave women in history: Eleanor Roosevelt, Florence Nightingale, Madame Curie, Corrie ten Boom, Amelia Earhart, Marie Antoinette. *Okay, maybe not the last one.*

I'll get through this. I'm not losing my vision or my hearing. I'm not losing my ability to walk, to hug, to communicate. I'm not facing the guillotine before an angry mob or hiding in a cupboard as Nazis ransack my apartment. I'm not injecting myself with an experimental Ebola vaccine.

I pick up the Churchill biography and keep re-reading the same few pages, unable to concentrate. Aware of a sudden sticky warmth between my legs, I scurry to the bathroom in my hospital gown and anti-slip socks. *Arrgh, just my luck! An unexpected visit from Aunt Flo.*

I hadn't expected this, but I'd packed my suitcase for that contingency. After my diagnosis, Dr. Point Guard advised me to stop taking birth control pills in case the cancer was estrogen-positive, so my body is oblivious to any calendar. I peek out of the bathroom and flag down a nurse, asking if they have any sanitary supplies.

She shakes her head "no."

Unbelievable! The surgical suites are equipped with state-of-the-art medical equipment, scalpels, syringes, plastic tubes, bandages of all sizes. But not one tampon or maxipad!

Like every woman at least once in her life, I improvise a temporary fix and return to my cubicle. "I need my suitcase," I tell Ryan.

"I thought you wouldn't need it until after…"

"*Now.* I need it *now!*" He looks dumbfounded, but goes to retrieve it.

While Ryan's in the parking lot, the anesthesiologist walks in. She is a petite, pretty brunette with tortoiseshell eyeglasses.

"I'm glad you're here," I say. "I'm ready for happy hour."

She laughs, shaking her head. "Not much longer."

I answer a litany of questions, confirming my identity yet again and relaying my previous experience with anesthesia. Finally, she brings in the magic syringe and injects it into my IV. *Ahhh.* I've been a tangle of nerves all morning.

"Don't worry, we'll take good care of you." She turns to leave, then pauses, noticing my Churchill biography. "Good book?"

"Very."

"Never, never, never give up!" she declares, exiting the cubicle. "I'll be back soon."

Within minutes, my body feels boneless. Things are starting to get fuzzy around the edges. Soon, this ordeal will be over.

Disconcertingly, Aunt Flo is becoming a demanding houseguest. When Ryan returns with my suitcase, I grab some supplies. The nurses don't want me walking around after the sedative, so I peek out from behind the curtain. When the coast is clear, I dash to the bathroom.

Within a few seconds, the lavatory looks like a crime scene from CSI, with scarlet splatters on the toilet, wall, and floor.

Enough already! How unlucky can I be? Having a mastectomy is bad enough, but dealing with the worst period of my life on the same day? Is this Mother Nature's sick practical joke?

Too embarrassed to tell anyone my predicament, I stumble to my knees in my hospital gown, the IV line dragging behind me, and scrub the bathroom floor with antibacterial soap and wadded-up paper towels. (Okay, maybe HazMat inspectors would disapprove of my clean-up efforts, but I don't have any blood-borne pathogen, so no harm, no foul!)

I stagger back toward my cubicle, embarrassed to see Rock Star Surgeon, already wearing his surgical cap, cooling his heels.

Ryan meets me in the hallway. "What took you so long?" he stage-whispers. "They've been waiting."

"Sorry," I mumble to the crowd surrounding my cubicle. I climb onto my gurney and take a deep breath.

Suddenly Pop is there, too, standing by Ryan as I'm wheeled away.

Everything is softer, slightly blurry, the pre-operative sedative soothing my nerves.

Medical experts say that when someone loses consciousness, hearing is the last sense to go. Nurses advise you not to say anything in front of an unconscious person that you wouldn't want overheard. But in my case, the last remaining sense seems to be my inappropriate and wacky sense of humor. Cancer can take away a lot of things, but it can't touch that.

"No more wet t-shirt contests for me!" I joke as I'm rolled into the operating room.

(Note to Mom: I've never, ever entered a wet t-shirt contest. I promise.)

Surrounded by people in surgical scrubs. I blink from the bright overhead lights.

"We're starting anesthesia now," a voice announces.

I turn my head toward the wall stacked to the ceiling with

metal cabinets and drawers.

"Doesn't look like on TV," I mumble. "*ER* or *Grey's Anatomy.*"

"Relax," Rock Star Surgeon says. "Count along with me."

"Umm, I'm still awake. Don't think the anesthesia is work..."

Divine Secret: You can do this!

Repeat after me: I can do this, I can do this, I can do this, I can do this, I can do this, I can do this, I can do this, I can do this, I can do this, I can do this, I can do this, I can do this, I can do this, I can do this...

He leans down close to me, taking my hand and looking into my eyes.

Oh, how sweet, I think. He's soooo niiiiiiiiiiicccccccccceeeee...

Treatment:

Whacking Cancer with My Handbag

Seeing My Battle Scars

August 2007

I hear beeps. Muffled conversations. Part of me wants to drown them out, to sink back into sweet unawareness.

"She's waking up!" I recognize Mom's voice.

I'm in the recovery room. *It's over.*

Closing my eyes, I give in to the grogginess, which lures me like a sea nymph.

Yet squeaking gurney wheels intrude. Louder, closer chirps and hums of medical equipment. Scattered comments.

"Hello!" Someone is nudging my shoulder.

"You're waking up." A brisk yet pleasant voice. *Nurse, probably.*

"Honey?" I hear Ryan.

I blink against the light.

"Surgery's done." He reaches for my hand. "Everything went well."

Mom strokes my hair. "Hey, sweetie. How do you feel?"

"Not great. Too hot." I'm not hurting much, but I'm burning up, cocooned in stiff, heavy blankets.

They loosen the linens and fan me with magazines.

Oppressed by the heat, I'm pummeled with nausea. I lurch upward, afraid I'll have to dash to the bathroom. A wave of pain rolls through my chest and arm.

"Hold on," the nurse warns me. "I don't want you getting up yet. I'll bring you more anti-nausea meds." She returns in a few minutes, handing me an iced soda to settle my stomach, along with a plastic basin—just in case.

"This should help." She holds out a tiny paper cup containing a pill. I swallow the medicine.

"I heard your nodes look clean." The nurse gives me an encouraging smile.

"That's what the surgeon told me," Ryan confirms.

My mom chimes in. "That's great news!"

"We can't be sure until the pathology report comes back," my husband explains. "But it looks good."

I nod, as a heavy veil of apprehension lifts. Important news, but I'm too muddle-headed to respond.

As the queasy sensation subsides, I feel a throbbing achiness under my armpit, but no searing pain. With the blankets peeled back, I allow myself a quick glance at my chest, noticing the lack of symmetry underneath the surgical bandages.

Although I knew what operation was planned, my heart sinks as I look at the area where my breast used to be. Thinking about having a mastectomy was one thing; seeing the vacant area on my chest makes the cancer undeniable.

My eyes dart away, unwilling to linger on this particular visual. I don't want to look closely or think too much. I'd rather stay in this loopy haze, like I've downed a pitcher of margaritas without any chips and salsa.

I drift in and out of sleep, tuning out the bright overhead lights and beeping monitors.

The nurse pushes my gurney to another area of the recovery ward. "Sorry, but your room's not ready yet," she explains.

The hospital is overbooked?

I try to read one of the magazines Mom fanned me with earlier, but I can't concentrate. Instead, I watch the nurses flit around the room, tending to their patients.

∼

Several hours later, as the clock ticks on, we are still stuck in recovery.

Mom goes home to make dinner for the kids and oversee homework. After running out of supportive things to say, Ryan gets out his laptop. There are no televisions in the post-op area, probably because the patients here, still groggy, aren't that cognizant of their surroundings.

To pass the time, I start up conversations with the nurses, asking random questions whenever one walks by.

"Somebody's still feeling the Versed," one nurse stage-whispers to another, tilting her head in my direction.

Finally, an orderly pushes my gurney out of the recovery room, the staff relieved to say goodbye to their Chatty Cathy patient.

I feel a touch of freedom as I'm wheeled into my hospital room, but that is quickly stifled when a nurse introduces herself and wraps my legs with weird inflatable encumbrances.

"What are those things?"

"Air compression leg wraps. To prevent blood clots."

She velcros plastic around both my legs, and turns on the machine. With a loud hum, the wraps inflate.

They sort of remind me of the water wings Larissa wears in the pool to stay afloat. Except that these leg things are ginormous, lacking any recreational vibe.

After a few minutes, the compression wraps make another noise as they deflate with a whoosh, then inflate again in a rhythmic manner. Now I'm not just attached to an IV line, I'm physically anchored to the bed.

The nurse instructs me in the use of the pain pump, explaining that the medicine is released at timed intervals to keep patients from self-administering too high a dosage.

I give the button an inaugural push. An analgesic haze might be a pretty good thing, a way to postpone ruminating about cancer. I glance at the clock and try to estimate how many minutes I must wait before getting another squirt of morphine.

Before she leaves, the nurse writes "Committed to Service Excellence" on a whiteboard and adds her name. Then the nursing aide and custodian stop by, introducing themselves and scribbling their names with a felt marker. The nursing aide explains she'll be checking my vitals and responding to the call button. The custodian will change bed sheets and empty my trash can.

Soon after, the food services lady arrives to deliver the dinner tray to my rolling bedside table. There's green jello and a cardboard cup of melting ice cream, but the entrée is hidden under a plastic cover.

Adding her name to the whiteboard, she looks me in the eye and says, "I just want you to know—"

"That you're committed to *Service Excellence!*"

"Why, yes." She giggles.

"Lucky guess."

After she leaves the room, I lift the dome from my plate. *Hmm, some sort of gravy-laden mystery meat.* Seems they could use a touch of "Service Excellence" in the culinary department, perhaps some cooking tips from Bobby Flay or Rachael Ray.

I'm a little hungry, but nothing on the tray appeals.

Ryan stands up. "I'll go get something from the cafeteria so we can eat together."

"No fair. You get to choose and I'm stuck with jailhouse grub."

"Want me to bring you something back?"

"Please."

As he leaves, I push the morphine button. The cuisine may not merit five Michelin stars, but the pain pump is top-notch!

Ryan returns with large deli sandwiches, plus some fruit and two cookies. I eat part of my sandwich and a banana.

After dinner, the next shift of hospital personnel arrives. They introduce themselves and share another "Service Excellence" spiel.

Ryan spends the night in my room, sleeping in a vinyl recliner. He gets a little grumpy when I wake him up every hour. But I need him to unplug me from the inflatable leg casings so I can hobble to the bathroom. I can't help it; these IV lines keep top-ping me off with liquid.

~

Early the next morning, Ryan goes home to shower.

I'm drifting back to sleep when Rock Star Surgeon arrives.

*Why is it that the doctor **never** shows up during the 23 hours of the day that your family sits anxiously by your bedside awaiting a medical update? Hospital rounds inevitably coincide with the exact moment your loved ones dash out for coffee, a jaunt to the gift shop, or a quick trip home.*

Rock Star Surgeon is telling me something, but I'm having a hard time following. I'm fixated on the purple silk around his neck. "I really like your tie," I mumble.

"Thanks."

"That is one good-looking tie!"

"Okay." I hear a bit of irritation creeping into his voice. Maybe I'm getting too enamored with my pain pump.

"Let's take a look." He peels away the bandage to reveal a long, reddish gash stitched together with black, wiry thread. I push back the grogginess and take a quick peek. The skin looks a tad reddish-brown at one end of the scar.

"Did you, uh, miss something? That dark area...isn't that part of my nipple?"

"No, that's where the suture ends. Your incision looks fine," he explains. "We talked about this already. Remember? I told you that I don't do nipple-sparing mastectomies because I think it's too risky to leave that tissue behind."

"Uh, okay." Normally, I'd be put off by his exasperated demeanor, but I'm feeling quite mellow. *Maybe I should buy Ryan a purple tie.*

The doctor scribbles something on my chart and exits my room.

Rock Star Surgeon has left the building!

~

After breakfast, Pastor Barry shows up for a visit. I'm glad to
see him, but self-conscious about my appearance, so I clutch a
small pillow to my chest. We don't talk much about cancer or
illness. Instead, I ask about how he met his wife, his experiences
serving on a navy submarine, and favorite places he's traveled.

Ryan returns and joins the conversation until Barry leaves.
Then he turns on his laptop and we update my *CaringBridge*
page. The morning is filled with floral deliveries and more
bowls of green jello, since lunch is generally served at 10:30 a.m.
Hospital Standard Time.

Medical staffers check my vitals on a frequent basis. They
take my temperature, measure my heart rate, and replace my
empty IV bags. Sometimes I joke with them about the "excellent" way they just checked my blood pressure. They also make
me breathe into a spirometer, a plastic contraption that whistles
and measures my lung output, helping fend off pneumonia.

One of the nurses teaches us how to clear the icky surgical
drains using a pinch and slide motion. The technique moves
the fluid along the plastic tubing into collection bulbs shaped
like tiny grenades. I feel like a squid with my tangle of rubbery
appendages.

It's early afternoon— the perfect nap time—so why am I surprised when the next shift of personnel stops by to introduce
themselves? And while I'm glad they're "Committed to Service
Excellence," I should tell them I don't need my trashcan emp-
tied at 5 a.m.

~

That evening, Mom brings the kids for a visit. I don't want them
scared by my appearance. Before they arrive, I ask the nursing
aide to temporarily unplug me from my IV and help me put
on a fresh camisole with pockets to hide the drain bulbs. My
scar is tender, but I stuff a lightweight polyester puff into the
right side. It looks ridiculous, in no way disguising my missing breast, so I try to cover the asymmetry with a loose-fitting

green chenille bed jacket.

I've just put away my lipstick when the kids walk into the room. They seem nervous, their eyes downcast.

"Mommy!" wails Larissa. "Are you okay?"

"I'm fine, sweetie."

At my bedside, I give them each an awkward hug with my unaffected left arm. The boys make skittish eye contact with me, not sure where to look or what to say.

"Hey, guys," I joke. "Staying in the hospital isn't so bad. I get to read and watch TV all day. No grocery shopping, no laundry, no cooking."

"Mom's going to be fine," Ryan reassures them. "Her surgery went great."

"I'll be home in another day or two," I add. "Then Dad gets to play nursemaid while you guys have fun on the cruise with your aunts and uncles."

"I'm the nursemaid?"

"Why, yes! Didn't you see the bell Justine gave me to keep on the nightstand? You'd better expect a lot of ringing!" Semi-serious, my girlfriend had told me to use the bell when I needed something.

The kids start laughing, and Mom shows us the birthday cake she prepared in Nick's honor.

"I remember the last time I ate birthday cake in the hospital." I smile at my younger son. "The nurse brought one to my room on the day you were born."

"Was I there?" Alex asks.

"Yes," Ryan explains. "I took you to see Mom and your new brother."

"You were only three years old and not that interested in Nick," I tell him. "But you did have a great time playing with the controls for my hospital bed, making it raise and lower. Up-down, up-down."

The kids laugh. Then, we sing "Happy Birthday" and watch Nick open gifts I'd purchased and wrapped in advance. We eat chocolate cake and talk about the family cruise. Once again,

I'm grateful that my sister-in-law has offered to chaperone the boys. The house will be a much quieter place for a few days.

~

Ryan spends a second night in the recliner, but heads home the next morning after Mom arrives to help with the discharge process.

We're figuring out the logistics of how to load floral arrangements into her car when Rock Star Surgeon stops by. He seems pleased I'm more lucid, weaned off the pain pump. After a cursory look at my incision, he jots down a date and time for my follow-up appointment and makes notes on his clipboard.

"How are you feeling?"

"Not too bad. I'm surprised the pain hasn't been worse."

"I use a lot of local anesthetic in the OR. My patients say it helps diminish discomfort."

"Much appreciated!" I add, "Can I take the pain pump home? As a souvenir, like the socks and the plastic breathing gadget?"

Rock Star Surgeon shakes his head, bemused. Maybe he's not used to my level of wackiness in the post-surgical ward.

"As I told your family earlier," he continues, "based on what we saw in your sentinel node biopsy, it appears all of your lymph nodes are cancer-free."

This is hugely reassuring, indicating the cancer was contained within my breast and unlikely to have spread anywhere else. Finding malignant cells in the sentinel nodes would require another operation—an axillary node dissection—to remove many more lymph nodes. Also, with cancer in the nodes, chemotherapy would likely be mandatory, not optional.

"We can't be completely sure until the full pathology report comes back," Rock Star Surgeon continues. "Yet sentinel node biopsy is pretty reliable. The average error rate is ten percent. But mine is only five percent."

I smile and nod. "That's good to hear."

After he leaves the room, Mom and I burst into school-girl

giggles. I deepen my voice and dust off an imaginary lapel, mimicking his words, "The average error rate is ten percent, but mine is only five percent!"

Mom shakes her head. "Poor guy doesn't have much confidence, does he?"

"Hey, a little ego is a good thing for a surgeon."

"I hear the best are like fighter pilots—cocky and sure of themselves."

"I'm cool with that. Don't want any insecure surgeon cutting on me!"

Laughing, Mom leaves to get the car while I finish dressing. A nurse comes in to remove my IV, ripping the tape from my arm in a most excellent fashion.

~

I'm alone, finally disconnected from all medical apparatus. The room is silent, devoid of beeps and whooshes.

Time to face the mirror.

I've taken fleeting glances at my scar when Rock Star Surgeon or one of the nurses peeked inside my camisole, but haven't worked up the nerve for a good, long look. I stand in front of the mirror, the one place I've avoided in my tiny hospital room. My heart is thumping and my nerves are jittery.

Lifting up my surgical camisole, I utter an involuntary gasp. The right side of my chest is flattened, a thin strip of surgical tape stretched across folds of flesh.

I feel dizzy and unnerved, cringing at my unfamiliar reflection. I really am dealing with cancer, my body a battlefield showing the collateral damage.

My throat tightens. I swallow a sob. Some days my diagnosis seemed surreal, more like a disjointed nightmare. Assuming I was in good health, I'd been caught off guard, stunned by the news of malignancy. But there's no denying it now.

Looking away, I take a few deep breaths, reminding myself that many Pink Sisters have been in my shoes. I'm not the only woman who's had to work up the courage to view cancer's malicious signature scrawled across her body. I force myself to face the mirror again.

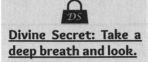

Divine Secret: Take a deep breath and look.

I know it's scary, but take a deep breath and look in the mirror. Go ahead and cry. Then, a little later, look again. You do not look like Frankenstein's monster. Your scars will fade from angry red to a subtle silvery-pink. You are still you, still beautiful, with or without your breasts.

My reflection *is* shocking, but not as scary as I'd feared. Looking at some post-mastectomy pictures on the Internet gave me an idea of what to expect. *Thank God for Pink Sisters who bravely shared their photos!*

But my appearance differs from the women shown with skin pulled taut across their chests. Since Rock Star Surgeon did a skin-sparing procedure, I have folds of flesh, like a deflated balloon, on the right side of my chest. Saddened by my loss of invincibility as much as by the loss of my breast, I cry.

Separating the Princes
from the Frogs

O n the drive home, I tuck a small pillow between the
seat belt and my tender chest. Three days ago, as a nervous pledge of the Pink Sorority, I'd left for the hospital in pre-dawn darkness. Today, on a hot, sunny afternoon, I
return home a fully-initiated member.

Maybe someday I'll consider my scars marks of honor, like
the carvings on the face of a young Maori warrior, proving
affiliation and kinship. But for now they remind me only of
disease and loss.

When I walk into the house, everything looks the same,
yet different. I've only been gone for two nights, but it feels
more like two years. As Mom and Ryan bring my suitcase
and floral arrangements inside, I stand at the kitchen counter and open a stack of greeting cards, touched by the kind
messages.

In a few hours, it's time to measure and empty the fluid col-
lected in my four surgical drains. Mom offers to help with this
yucky task.

Ryan shakes his head. "No, I want to do it!"

Surprised and skeptical, I look at him. "You're kidding, right?
You don't do blood and gore."

"No, I'm serious."

In the delivery room for Alex, Ryan almost passed out, a nurse catching him before he hit his head on a stainless steel table. Over the years, whenever a kid has needed stitches, I was the one cleaning the wound and driving to the ER.

Yet, because he wants to help—in a tangible, task-oriented way—Ryan shoulders the icky drain routine. Maybe the scientist in him views it as a lab experiment, regarding my bodily fluids as just another chemical solution. I don't understand how he gets past his squeamishness to do this, but for me, it's sweeter than a box of Godiva chocolates.

Granted, Ryan's a practical engineer who considers efficiency next to godliness. He doesn't ride to my rescue on a white stallion like Fabio in a pirate shirt—or more to my taste, Mark Wahlberg in no shirt—but he's my prince nonetheless. Like most guys, he doesn't have much patience for the empathetic listening thing, but give him a dragon to slay and he'll spring into action.

~

With the boys on the cruise and Larissa at a play date, the house is unusually quiet. I rest on the couch, soaking up the tranquility, reminding myself that for someone with cancer, I'm pretty damn lucky. I feel safe and protected, blanketed in a cloud of love and friendship.

The pain is manageable as long as I remain relatively still, my side and underarm area aching more than my chest. I try to keep my right arm slightly elevated on a stack of pillows to minimize swelling. One of the pillows is almost too beautiful to use for such a utilitarian task. Edged with lace and pink embroidery, it's a gift from Mary Lou's mother back in Texas, a lovely woman with cheekbones that could scrape the ice off your windshield.

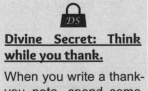

Divine Secret: Think while you thank.

When you write a thank-you note, spend some time thinking of the giver's kind gesture and the healing power of love and friendship.

Apparently, she could be the next Martha Stewart of medical supplies, helping Kmart shoppers recuperate in style.

I spend the time reading, watching DVDs, and napping. The house looks like a florist's shop, with blooms on every counter and tabletop. Each day brings more cards, inspirational jewelry, and home-cooked meals. The object of so much positive attention, I'm expecting Chris Harrison and Brooke Burke to crown me with a rhinestone tiara any minute now.

The downside is that sometimes I feel awkward and self-conscious about my appearance when a visitor drops by. My scar is still tender, and must heal for several more weeks before I can be fitted for a prosthetic. With the drains still attached, I can't even wear a soft sports bra.

Also, taking a shower requires ingenuity. It's too painful to let the surgical drains dangle free and risks opening the stitches, so I play MacGyver, removing the belt from my bathrobe, stringing it with the plastic bulbs, and then tying the contraption around my waist.

I dutifully perform the arm exercises prescribed in my recovery instructions folder, walking my hand up the shower wall like a crab. I'm not allowed to shave under my right arm, which bugs me, so I put on my imaginary beret and pretend I'm a French poet. Within a few days, my range of motion improves enough that I'm able to reach up and wash my hair, a task Mom had been doing for me in the kitchen sink.

Divine Secret: Consider restricting the visitor list.

Think about your personal comfort zone. Are you going to be self-conscious about your appearance right after surgery? You may want to consider limiting visitors to immediate family or close friends.

~

A week after surgery, Ryan drives me to Rock Star Surgeon's office for the follow-up appointment. Caring Nurse escorts us to the exam room, a big smile on her face.

"We've got some good news for you!" She hands me a hospital gown. "But I'm going to let the doctor tell you himself."

Moments later, Rock Star Surgeon breezes into the room, shaking our hands. "Your pathology report is back," he crows. "All nodes are clean."

"That's great!" Ryan's face lights up.

"I'm so relieved." *It's official!*

"Me, too," the doctor replies. "And since your cancer hasn't spread to the nodes, you might not need chemo. There's a test called *Oncotype* that helps predict your risk of recurrence and whether chemo would be beneficial."

Maybe I should be relieved when he says this, but my insides quiver like the green hospital jello. I don't *want* chemo, but I'm determined to do whatever I can to ward off recurrence.

However, I do recall Dr. Point Guard explaining that *Oncotype* analyzes numerous genes from a patient's tumor sample. I'm not sure how I feel about a lab test deciding whether I receive chemo, but I should take these personalized results into account. Even if my treatment path is yet to be determined, an official report of clean nodes is very positive news—definitely something to celebrate!

Rock Star Surgeon examines my scar and reviews the chart documenting my drain output. "You are healing nicely. We can take one drain out today, but you need to keep the others in a little longer."

"Really?"

"We don't want to remove them too early." He explains that fluid could collect in my chest, becoming a painful seroma, which would require needle aspiration.

Sigh. Guess I'll have to deal with my plastic tentacles a bit longer.

After Rock Star Surgeon bids us goodbye, Caring Nurse prepares for the procedure. She wipes the area with alcohol and snips the stitches holding the drain in place. "Okay, now exhale."

I feel a strange tugging sensation, but minimal pain, as she pulls out the tubing snaked through my body.

"How much longer until I can get the others out?"

"That depends. Call me when you see a significant decrease in drainage. Try taking it easy the next few days," she advises. "Too much activity can be counterproductive when you're trying to reduce the amount of fluid produced."

That night, with one less drain, it's easier to build myself a comfortable nest of pillows. I drift to sleep quickly but awaken in the middle of the night. I hear Ryan stirring.

"You awake?"

"Yeah." He moves closer, draping his arm around my waist.

"Good news today."

"Honey, it was great news."

We turn together for a kiss and cling to each other, our emotions intense and fragile.

I'm shy about my appearance. Nervous and tentative. But he touches my scar, gently, reverently, as if stroking a swath of velvet. My anxieties melt away. The camisole I'm wearing—constructed of loose, stretchy cotton with drain pockets—is nothing like the provocative, wench-like bustier you'd see on the cover of a romance novel. I'm lopsided, scarred, and pale, yet have never felt more loved.

Divine Secret: Help your partner help you.

It's likely your partner wants to help but doesn't know how. Give him (or her) something tangible to do, especially if he's not great in the "empathetic listening" department. Keep in mind that he's scared, too, and may not want to talk as much as you need to. Don't expect your partner to be comfortable in every support role; sometimes you need a close friend or Pink Sister.

My Chemical Romance

Tonight is a big night for the Chapman residence—school open house. Alex is starting high school, Nick will be at the middle school, and Larissa is heading to kindergarten. I'm glad that I shopped for basic school supplies, including Larissa's all-important backpack, before surgery. My incision is not as tender, but I still have the drains, so I wear my softest, loosest bra, stuffed with socks on the right side, underneath my baggiest shirt. I tuck the drain bulbs into the waistband of my khaki capris, hoping to conceal them.

We go to the elementary school first. I can still remember Alex's very first day, when I took a picture of him at the front door with his backpack, wearing cargo shorts and a Winnie-the-Pooh t-shirt. Milling in the school corridors, Larissa is excited to see her neighborhood friends and meet her teacher, a young woman with a sweet demeanor. As Larissa checks out the activity centers for reading, puzzles, and Lego play, I pull the teacher aside.

"Did the counselor fill you in? Tell you I'm being treated for cancer?"

"Yes," she says. "Don't worry, I'll give your daughter extra hugs and attention."

I do feel awkward at Larissa's school because we see some

friends and neighbors. I can sense them taking surreptitious looks at my post-surgical chest, as if Rock Star Surgeon inserted an ocular magnet.

At the middle school, we walk through Nick's schedule and visit each classroom. Changing classes, memorizing locker combinations, dressing out for gym—all new and different experiences for him.

The high school seems a bit big and intimidating, but Alex is happy to see his friends in the hallways, where they compare notes about teachers assigned and electives chosen. The majority of teens here with their parents appear to be freshmen or sophomores, but occasionally I see a male upperclassman sprouting facial hair, appearing more adult than child. Only four years until Alex graduates and goes off to college.

So many milestones still ahead for my kids.

~

About three weeks after my mastectomy, Ryan and I go to the first "official" appointment with Dr. Point Guard. To disguise the drains and obvious asymmetry, I wear a blousy short-sleeved cardigan.

Dr. Point Guard greets me with a gentle hug and escorts us to a small conference room. I'm eager to hear his treatment recommendations.

"I'm sorry, but I don't have your *Oncotype* results back yet." He explains that the pathology lab didn't send a large enough tissue sample, so he's re-ordered the test.

Not again.

I wince in annoyance. *Yes, lab techs are human, mistakes happen, yadda, yadda, yadda. But why do they keep screwing up MY tissue samples?* I'd been anxious to hear the test score calculating the odds that, within the next ten years, the disease would return—not to my left breast, or the tiny remnants of tissue remaining after surgery on the right, but as Stage IV cancer, metastasized to my bones or other organs.

"Don't worry," Dr. Point Guard assures me. "We have enough information to discuss options—at least hypothetically—until we get your results. There's an online program, *Adjuvant Online*, doctors used prior to *Oncotype* to help determine the risk versus benefit."

He explains that in the past, tumor size was used as the main factor for determining the need for chemotherapy, but these days treatment is becoming much more customized.

Since we don't know whether I'll be identified as having a low, intermediate, or high risk of recurrence, we discuss the positives and negatives of chemo in general.

"Chemo is not appropriate or advisable for certain people. It's not without risk of serious side effects," he explains. "With some of the most commonly-used chemo agents, there's about a two percent chance of developing heart failure and a one percent chance of developing leukemia from the treatment. If your risk of recurrence is already very low—let's say three to five percent—we might decide chemo isn't advisable for the small increment of potential benefit."

I consider this. Plenty of people have given me their unsolicited opinions about chemotherapy, some warning me not to do it, others encouraging me to go forth.

"Also," Dr. Point Guard continues, "since your cancer is estrogen- and progesterone-positive, you will benefit from tamoxifen, a drug that reduces your risk of recurrence."

"That's good."

Tamoxifen is often prescribed to pre-menopausal women for an extended period, significantly reducing recurrence, but I've read it can have side effects, such as increased risk of endometrial cancer and blood clots. Some Pink Sisters taking the medication have complained about slow, fuzzy thinking and newly-acquired "tamoxiflab," an extra layer of pudge around their midsection.

But I'm not going to let the possibility of that happening bring me down. Perhaps tamoxifen will make me even more clueless and chubby, but hey, it's still better than another round of breast cancer.

Dr. Point Guard goes over the AJCC (American Joint Committee on Cancer) Guidelines, the "Treatment Bible" for oncologists. He explains that I have Stage I cancer with neither node involvement nor spread of malignant cells beyond my breast. Until recently—since the survival rate for patients with early-stage breast cancer is very good—doctors have used tumor size as the main indicator for recommending chemo. Generally, for a tumor of one centimeter or less, chemo was not advised.

Okay, but I have two tumors: one centimeter and seven millimeters. What does this mean for me?

"She doesn't need chemo?" Ryan's expression brightens.

"I discuss pros and cons with all my patients."

"What about the fact I had two tumors?"

Dr. Point Guard explains that, according to the AJCC, staging is done by the size of the largest tumor, not the cumulative tumor load. In my case, staging is for the one centimeter tumor, not the cumulative 1.7 centimeters.

"I've heard this before, but it makes me uncomfortable." *How can I ignore the presence of a second tumor? If they'd gone undetected and untreated, would the two separate malignancies have merged into one giant, evil mass?*

As a rabid Internet researcher, I tell the doctor I've read medical journal abstracts indicating not all oncologists agree with the AJCC on this issue.

"I understand your concern," replies Dr. Point Guard, "but that's what the data is showing us. Official guidelines recommend using largest tumor size for staging—not the cumulative size. Yet, as you've noted, there's some controversy."

Why can't anything about this stupid disease be definitive?

"I'm considered young for diagnosis, right?"

"Yes. As we discussed earlier, cancer tends to be more aggressive in younger women. That's one factor to consider. We also look at the tumor's grade. According to our lab reports, yours was rated moderately aggressive."

Great. One more in-between, mediocre factor to weigh! If the cancer was deemed slow-growing and indolent, I might be comfortable skipping chemo. If it was labeled aggressive, then I would have no doubts about chemo being a wise choice.

What I feel now is confused!

"I'll call you the minute I get your score. In the meantime, I'll introduce you to the nurse who teaches my patients about chemotherapy. We'll set up some time for you to talk."

~

As we walk to the car, my mind is spinning.

"What are you thinking?" Ryan asks.

I sigh and shake my head in frustration. "I don't know."

"Finding out your *Oncotype* score will help."

"I'm not happy about the delay. I expected to make the decision today."

We cross the parking lot, our footsteps thudding on the concrete.

"On one hand, I'm early-stage, with no spread to nodes. And I'm hormone-positive, which means I can take medication to help prevent recurrence."

"All good."

"I know some people in my shoes would forgo chemo, and that would be a reasonable decision," I explain "But a few other factors make me favor chemo: my age, the fact that the cancer was graded moderately aggressive and—in my mind at least—the presence of more than one tumor."

"Chemo can be rough. But I want you around for a long, long time."

Ryan opens the passenger door, and I slide inside. He puts the key in the ignition but doesn't start the engine.

"Yeah, so unless I get a super-low *Oncotype* score, I'm going to do chemotherapy. My Stage IV scare—when it looked like cancer had spread to my lungs—was a definite tipping point. That was scary!"

Ryan nods, resigned. "I never want to go through that again."

One factor—that I can't examine under a microscope or quantify—is my peace of mind. *If I skip chemotherapy, how will I feel if the cancer comes back?*

~

Back home, I dig out my pathology report. In the corner of the page, in a teeny, tiny font, is the name and phone number of the doctor who examined my malig-

Divine Secret: It's your body. You get to be the "Decider."

Choosing a treatment path can be confusing and difficult. Work in partnership with your medical providers. Educate yourself, ask lots of questions, weigh the pros and cons. Then choose the option that seems right for you.

nant cells. Frankly, I suspect pathologists are anti-social types, preferring the sterile elegance of their microscopes to the messiness of living, breathing patients.

I frown. This is the second time I've had an issue with this lab.

Forget my complaints about the hospital food service's mystery meat. If any department needs to show a little more "Service Excellence," it's Pathology.

Emboldened by frustration, I dial the number and a lady doctor picks up.

"Hello," I say, trying to maintain a sweet Southern tone behind gritted teeth. "Sorry to bother you. You probably don't receive many calls from patients."

"Uh, no. Not really."

I tell her my name and explain the situation. "I'm being treated for breast cancer, but your lab didn't send enough tissue out for my *Oncotype* test. So my results are delayed."

"I'm sorry that happened. We've already sent out another tumor sample."

"This isn't the first issue I've had with you guys. After my biopsy, someone forgot to do the ER/PR testing."

"My apologies," the doctor says. "I know we've placed a 'rush' request on your *Oncotype* result, so hopefully you'll hear something soon."

"Okay, thanks."

The doctor sounds so humble on the phone that I feel a little guilty for chewing her out. But just a *little*.

~

I'm very curious about what my *Oncotype* score will tell me. But who decides where a number falls on the spectrum of low, moderate, or high? And how do they determine where to draw a line in the sand delineating these groups?

I call Teal Ribbon Mom; I have so many questions about chemo. Her voicemail picks up, so I leave a message, hoping she'll call back.

In the weeks since surgery, my discomfort has declined and my range of motion has improved. After being mostly housebound for a month, I start driving again.

Divine Secret: Multidisciplinary tumor boards can offer a second opinion.

If you need help deciding on a treatment path, remember that many hospitals hold weekly tumor board meetings, where a team of oncologists, radiologists, surgeons, pathologists, nurse navigators, and social workers meet to discuss patient cases and make treatment recommendations.

All my drains are gone. My scar has healed enough that I can don a sports bra stuffed with a few soft socks. Adding another baggy shirt, I head to the Boobtique to be measured for my prosthesis.

I feel shy undressing, but Red-Headed Saleslady puts me at ease. "Dearie, I've been a certified fitter for decades. No need to feel embarrassed."

Soothed by her chatty and vivacious manner, I relax. After all, she's probably seen more topless ladies than Hugh Hefner.

Red-Headed Saleslady brings an assortment of breast forms into my dressing room so we can find the best fit. After trial and error, she decides they don't have my perfect clone in stock. She tells me it will have to be ordered but shouldn't take long to arrive.

I'm so sick of wearing these dowdy, baggy shirts, trying—without much success—to hide my post-surgical shape. *I would love to burn them all in a bonfire!*

~

A few days later, I stuff one side of my sports bra and drive to a small town having the odd distinction of three wig shops residing within a few short blocks. One downside to chemotherapy is the probable hair loss—particularly troublesome for someone raised in Texas, where big hair is a birthright.

In the first store, the merchandise is displayed on Styrofoam heads kept behind glass counters. The wigs look high quality with modern, not matronly, cuts. An Asian couple—maybe Chinese, Korean, or Vietnamese—greets me.

"I'd like to see that one," I say, pointing to a cute layered style.

"No," the salesman says, shaking his head. "Not good for you!"

I'm taken aback. Never have I had a salesperson refuse to show me something. This can't be a cultural thing. While in China to adopt Larissa, salespeople gushed with enthusiasm if we showed the slightest interest. Also, as the mother of a Chinese girl, I never want to stereotype people based on ethnicity.

"Okaaaaay," I answer, surprised and a little annoyed. "How about that one?" I point to a slightly longer wig, streaked with golden highlights.

"No, not for you!"

This is getting strange. *Really strange.*

"This one for you," he says, pulling a puffy blonde bob off the shelf.

It's not the look I'm going for, but I humor him and try it on.

"That you! Best for you!" He smiles and nods, his head bobbing like one of those toy velveteen dogs placed on the dashboard of a car.

"Yes, look!" His wife hands me a mirror.

"It's nice, but I'd prefer something more layered."

Crazy Wig Salesman crosses his arms and gives me a stern glare. "I businessman. I know what look good!"

He's a small man, but his expression is intimidating.

"I'll come back later. With a friend."

I turn toward the door, but he blocks my exit. "No! No! Friend only confuse you! Listen to me. I businessman."

"Uh, thanks, anyway." I fake left, then run right, dashing out the door.

At the second wig shop, the prices are lower but the choices less stylish. Everything looks dated and bouffant, like what you'd see on an older lady wearing a loud silk caftan.

I proceed to the third wig shop, but quickly rule it out due to the distinct hooker vibe.

Just for the heck of it, I try on a metallic silver Cleopatra wig, thinking it might be crazy fun. Then I realize Ryan and the kids would be mortified.

Divine Secret: You get to pick your own wig.

You can choose a wig that matches your pre-cancer hairstyle, completely disguising your chemo-related hair loss. Or you can try on different styles and shades. Ever wanted to be a redhead? Or have curly hair? Here's your chance. You might prefer cute hats and colorful scarves. Or go au natural. Do whatever gives you confidence, lifts your spirits, and makes you the most comfortable!

Walking back to my car, I pause outside the window of the first shop.

Uh, oh! Big mistake.

Crazy Wig Salesman runs outside, a big grin on his face. "You back!" He stretches out his arm, like he's preparing for a hug. "You listen to me!"

"Sorry, not today." I zig backwards on the sidewalk and zag across the street, as if I'm a running back going for a "Hail Mary" pass. Then I duck into the bookstore, a place more in my comfort zone.

I'm Not a *Sex in the City* Girl

I attend a different support group meeting in a posh section of the city, just around the corner from the downtown cancer center. The demographics of the participants seem to skew younger and more affluent than the local hospital group with Faux-Hippie Facilitator and Cat Fanatic.

The ladies are friendly and welcoming. Judging from their bandannas or extremely short hair, I'm able to spot several women who are currently in—or have just finished—chemotherapy.

"Glad you're here," says one, asking me where I'm at in my cancer journey.

A second woman walks over and introduces herself. "Who's your breast surgeon?"

When I mention Rock Star Surgeon, they practically swoon.

"Oh, I just love him!"

"He was mine, too. He's wonderful!"

If there was a *Tiger Beat* magazine for survivors, Rock Star Surgeon would be on the cover.

After chatting awhile, I introduce myself to two women who appear to be in their 30s, both wearing batik-print scarves. They share their experiences with chemo and write down their names and phone numbers, encouraging me to call with questions.

The group's president walks to the podium, signaling it's time to find a seat. I reluctantly step away from the cheese chunks, fresh fruit, and cookies.

"Welcome, everyone," she says. "Do we have any newcomers tonight?"

I raise my hand. Looking around the room, I spot another woman with her hand in the air. She appears to be in her 70s and is accompanied by her husband, the only male in the room.

After a few announcements, the moderator introduces the speaker for tonight's agenda, a "sexology" expert.

Huh? There are colleges where you major in sex? In an academic—rather than recreational—way?

Apparently so.

Taking the microphone, a bubbly brunette divulges her impressive credentials. She wastes no time jumping headfirst into her subject, asking questions that inspire oversharing. "How often do you ladies reach orgasm?"

As audience members disclose their personal batting averages, I slide down in my chair. One woman recommends specific sex toys she uses to "rev" herself up for her spouse.

Sexology Expert decides the comments have provided a nice segue for "show and tell." She holds up a vibrator, touting the model's special features, before handing it to a woman in the front row.

Next, she holds up a premium model, espousing the variable angle settings. She turns it on for a demonstration. The vibrator rotates like a kinky hand-held blender.

"Oh, my!"

"Wow."

"That looks dangerous!"

The room erupts in laughter.

Sneaking furtive glances, I spot the red-faced older couple. Poor guy had no idea what he was walking into!

The lady beside me hands me a vibrator. I pass it on like I'm playing "hot potato."

Can I slip away without being noticed?

Over the years, I've received a few invitations to Pure Romance sex toy parties, similar to a Tupperware or Pampered Chef event, but with decidedly different merchandise. I've always declined and never regretted it. If my neighbors or colleagues are into fuzzy handcuffs or edible underwear, I'd rather not know.

"What other products do you find helpful?" Sexology Expert queries. "Any favorite brands of lubricant?"

"The old standard, K-Y!"

"Pjur!"

"Astroglide!" shouts the woman next to me.

My face turns as crimson and mottled as the strawberries on the fruit tray. I am *so* not Carrie Bradshaw. I'll never share a play-by-play of bedroom antics with my BFFs over brunch.

"Ladies," Sexology Expert asks, "how has treatment affected your libido and response?"

The question inspires honest feedback.

"I miss the feeling of touch on my breasts."

"That area is completely numb."

"It's hard to feel attractive, especially when shopping for a swimsuit or cocktail dress."

"I've been depressed since my diagnosis, never in the mood."

"I invest in nice lingerie, bubble baths, and manicures to help me feel feminine again."

"I avoid magazines because the photos remind me of what I've lost."

As I listen to my Pink Sisters share their experiences, I begin to rethink my discomfort with tonight's topic. There appears to be a trifecta of common sexual repercussions following breast cancer: 1) self-image issues, 2) numbness and loss of sensation after surgery, and 3) hormonal changes due to drug treatments and chemotherapy.

Some of the women are years past treatment, but their sexual issues linger. Suddenly, I understand that the conversation is not just about sex. It's about how cancer can disrupt your emotional and physical intimacy. About how you feel when you look in the mirror. About how you grieve for the way you once felt.

Divine Secret: You can ask a Ta-Ta sister ANYTHING.

No matter how personal or sensitive the question, you can always find a fellow survivor to give you an honest answer. Never worry about TMI (too much information) with a breast cancer sister.

"Ladies, it's possible you'll get some feeling back," one survivor confides. "You know those weird pains and itchy feelings long after surgery? Those are nerves regenerating. It's not like before cancer, but some of my numbness has disappeared."

Sexology Expert listens, nodding in approval. "That's encouraging news." She looks around the room. "Did anyone's doctor talk about sexual function after cancer? Ask you how things were in that department?"

The room falls silent. Not a single woman speaks up.

Hmm, maybe there's a need for "Sexologists" after all.

Resource: pureromance.com

This company is sort of like an X-rated Toys"R"Us! You can buy products online, which they promise to ship in discreet, unmarked packages.

Reign of the Clone

September 2007

I return to the Boobtique to pick up "the clone," the nickname I've dubbed my prosthetic breast.

"Well, hello!" chirps Red-Headed Saleslady. "We're going to get you fixed up today."

Carrying a small cardboard box and a collection of bras, she follows me into the fitting room. She opens the package, handing me the beige silicone mound. It's heavier than I expected, with a squishy texture.

"It's weighted," she explains, "so it doesn't ride up."

Good thing, since my socks-stuffed-in-sports-bra fix has given me the appearance of diagonal boobs a time or two.

Less shell-shocked than on my previous visit, I'm pleasantly surprised by the array of options available to women who delay reconstruction or choose to forego it. Breast forms come in a variety of shapes, sizes, and skin tones. You can order a prosthetic insert with a fake nipple attached or as a stick-on accessory. Also, there are lightweight waterproof choices designed for swimming and exercise. Even partial forms in graduated sizes for women who need to "fill in" an area after lumpectomy.

Red-Headed Saleslady takes a bra off the hanger and waits for me to undress.

I hesitate, still reluctant to face my reflection.

"Now, dearie," she croons, slipping the silicone triangle into one of the bra pockets. "I've been doing this for twenty years. No need to feel shy."

I unbutton my blouse and slip off my sports bra.

"Try this one."

She's holding out an enormous beige bra with thick straps and seamed cups. It looks dowdy, like something from an old Montgomery Ward catalog.

As I hold out my arms, she fastens the clasp.

"Lean forward, doll."

She adjusts my solitary breast into the left bra cup and tugs the clone in place.

"Stand up, sweetheart."

I look in the mirror. *Not too bad.* While I've never coveted geriatric-style lingerie, I admit the post-mastectomy bra and prosthesis conceal my missing breast.

Divine Secret: Research your medical benefits and other options.

Your insurance should cover the cost of your prosthetic breast inserts, plus at least one or two post-mastectomy bras. Some policies will pay for a "medically necessary cranial prosthesis," aka wig. No insurance? Check with your hospital and the local chapter of the American Cancer Society. They may have a lending closet.

From her position behind me, Red-Headed Saleslady grabs my hands, smashing my palms against the bra cups.

She has me feeling myself up! Could this be any more surreal and awkward?

"Can't tell a difference, can you?"

Actually, I can. Still, I appreciate her efforts in making me feel better.

I ask to try a different bra, a seamless and satiny one.

"You're going to love this," she confides, slipping it off the hanger. "It's just like that expensive Le Mystere brand Oprah wears."

Well, if it's good enough for Oprah, it's good enough for me!

After she explains that my insurance will cover the cost of several post-mastectomy bras—deemed a medical necessity—I select three bras off the rack and order two more. Wadding up my baggy blouse and shoving it in the shopping bag, I wear a t-shirt home, happy to dress more like my old self.

~

Mom comes a few days later. I'm still waiting for my *Oncotype* score, so we decide to browse an upscale wig salon. *It never hurts to be prepared!* Although there's a large selection, most styles are huge and puffy. I've read that most women get their wigs trimmed and shaped, so I keep that in mind.

A saleswoman greets us at the door.

"Welcome," she says, smiling at Mom. "Has any-one ever told you that you look just like Blythe Danner?"

Divine Secret: The tlcdirect.org catalog/website offers great bargains!

This catalog/website, produced by the American Cancer Society, offers reasonably priced breast forms, bras, camisoles, wigs, hats, scarves, and other prod-ucts. Also, unlike many shops, if you change your mind you can exchange or return. (This came in handy after the platinum blonde wig I'd ordered—hoping for a Marilyn Monroe vibe—looked like an albino squirrel napping on my head.)

"Why, thank you," Mom answers.

"Then I must be the spitting image of her lovely daughter, Gwyneth Paltrow."

It's a joke—I'm at least twenty years older, five inches shorter, and forty pounds heavier than the Hollywood darling—but no one laughs.

"I've got a screen test with Spielberg tomorrow."

"Uh," Humorless Saleslady stumbles for a response. "How about I show you around?"

She walks us through the store, pointing out different styles and price points. "Natural hair wigs are very nice, but they require a good bit of upkeep, needing to be washed and styled as often as you'd do for your own hair."

I notice the real hair wigs are quite pricey, too, starting around $600, up to $2,000.

"One of the benefits of a synthetic is easy care," she adds. "Wash it about once a week and let it air dry. Give it a good shake before you put it on and you're ready to go."

Easy care sounds good.

"One thing: you do have to be careful with a synthetic to keep it away from heat sources," Humorless Saleslady warns. "Don't get too close to a hot dryer, oven, or dishwasher. Your wig might singe."

A synthetic wig comes with a warning to avoid laundry, cooking, and dishwashing? Even better!

She explains that synthetic wigs can vary widely in price, but most of the ones in their store range from $100 to $250. She tells us medical insurance will sometimes pay if the doctor writes a prescription for a "cranial prosthesis."

My insurance, alas, will not.

I browse through the displays, noticing that at the other end of the store there's another customer trying on wigs. She's quite young, with ripped jeans and a teeny tank top that reveals the tramp stamp tattoo on the small of her back. Her surly companion, a guy wearing gangsta-style saggy shorts and several piercings, glares at her.

Divine Secret: No need to spend big $$$ on a natural hair wig.

Consider an easy-care synthetic. My favorite brand was Noriko, a line from Rene of Paris. I purchased "Sky" and even got compliments on my hair from strangers and acquaintances who didn't realize I was wearing a wig!

Out of the corner of my eye, I watch as she tries on a Tina Turner–like electric blue wig. "Maybe I should try that one," I whisper, nudging Mom.

"It's so you."

"It'd be fun to wear home, just for the reaction."

"They'd be horrified." We stifle giggles.

On the clearance shelf, I discover the wig I like best, a synthetic that's shinier and more stylish than my own hair. *And it's half-priced. I love me some clearance sales!* Anyway, I don't want to spend a fortune on a wig; I might prefer a hat or scarf at times.

The shop has a "no return" policy, so I ask Humorless Saleslady to hold my selection for a few days.

Divine Secret: Keep your fashionista style!

Check out turbandiva.com for unique, fashion-forward headwear with an uptown, bohemian vibe.

~

Next, Mom and I head to a beauty supply outlet. At a recent *Look Good, Feel Better* makeup session, I'd learned that I'd need disposable applicators during chemo to keep my cosmetics germ-free. I'd left with some great swag; the instructor gave everyone a giant goody bag filled with lip gloss, eyeliner, and lotions. Many ladies don't go to the class until they start losing hair or eyebrows and lashes. But I decided to be pro-active, because otherwise I might feel too yucky and depressed to bother. *Gotta pre-empt that downward cycle.*

Divine Secret: Ask your friends to throw you a "hat party."

If your BFFs are looking for ways to help, have them lift your spirits by showering you with gifts of silky scarves, fedoras, baseball caps, etc.

29

Tilt-A-Whirl at the Fair

It's a Friday night in September so, in an effort to make life seem normal and uphold a family tradition, we go to the county fair. We walk through the animal exhibits, admiring cute piglets and fluffy bunnies. We stand in line for the Ferris wheel and eat candied apples. After Alex and Nick have reached their limit for family togetherness, I give them permission to head to the roller coasters and scramblers while Ryan and I take Larissa to the kiddie ride area.

My cell phone vibrates. It's Dr. Point Guard, so I hand Ryan my lemonade and corn dog.

"Hi, Joanna," he says. "I'm still at the office. I just received your *Oncotype* score, so I wanted to call you right away."

"Hold on," I say. "I can barely hear you. Let me find a quieter spot."

Walking away from the midway, I step over a tangle of extension cords. I stand in the trailer storage area behind the blinking lights and tinny music.

I take a deep breath. "Okay, go ahead."

He tells me my score, a number falling on the borderline between low and intermediate risk.

Once again, I've fallen into what I consider a gray area.

Oncotype predicts I have an 11% chance of distant

recurrence—meaning Stage IV/metastatic breast cancer—
within the next 10 years if I decide to forego chemotherapy.

"I wish all my patients could get a low, single-digit score,"
says Dr. Point Guard. "But since you're open to chemo, the
score's not a bad place to be. I'm relieved you didn't get a high
score. Statistically, your odds for recurrence are still quite
low, yet high enough for the treatments to provide some benefit."

Dr. Point Guard explains that *Oncotype* scores are calculated with the assumption that ER+ and PR+ (hormone recep-
tor positive) patients would also be receiving adjuvant therapy.
This consists of a daily dose of tamoxifen or, for someone postmenopausal, an aromatase inhibitor, to reduce or stop hormone
production. He says in my case, adding chemo to the adjuvant
drug regimen might knock down my risk of recurrence from
11% to around 7%.

Some Ta-Ta Sisters might not think my *Oncotype* score is
high enough to justify chemotherapy. With the same information and statistics, they might come to a different conclusion in
weighing the risks and potential benefits. I would respect that
choice, because we all have to listen to medical advice, assess
the risks versus benefits, and then decide what's best for us as
individuals.

This, however, is my perspective: think of your long-standing
bunco group or book club with 10 to 12 members. Statistically,
an 11% chance would be like losing one of them within the next
decade. Not something I'd expect with a group of age thirty-
and forty-something ladies.

So, though you may scrutinize pages of pie charts and statistics, an un-quantifiable yet important factor in deciding on
treatment is your personal preference. You have to look at the
science and listen to your heart. I know chemo is not a walk
in the park. There's a risk of serious long-term or life-threatening side effects. Yet, if I opted not to do chemo and the cancer returned, I'd kick myself with regret. I want to see my kids
grow up; I'm willing to do whatever I can to improve my odds.

From that perspective, a couple months of feeling crummy and losing my hair is not too high a price to pay.

"Yes," I say. "Let's do the chemo."

After Dr. Point Guard ends our conversation, I turn off my cell and put it in my purse. I walk back to the midway, where Ryan stands next to the mini-teacup ride while Larissa shrieks with delight. He looks at me, the question plastered on his face. "What did he say?"

"My score is borderline between low and moderate, but it's high enough for me to want the chemo."

He sighs. I know he's worried, but will support my choice.

I'll admit I'm scared, no doubt traumatized by a cheesy 70s movie featuring John Denver's "Sunshine on my Shoulders" as the theme song. The film featured a hippie chick who stopped cancer treatment, deciding death was preferable to nonstop upchucking. But I remind myself I endured serious bouts of morning sickness with Alex and Nick, keeping airline barf bags in my car.

Chemo may add only a few percentage points in my favor, but hopefully, it will mean that I never have to face a Stage IV diagnosis.

Walking through the fairgrounds in a daze, I barely notice the spinning lights. Game barkers shout, families laugh with glee, but I feel detached. I plaster a smile on my face, but my insides are quiet and solemn, the polar opposite of carnival merriment.

Divine Secret: Respect your Pink Sisters' treatment choices.

Many times there's not just one "right" answer when it comes to treating breast cancer; there may be several reasonable choices. Take the risks of serious side effects into account, but don't fear the treatment more than the disease. Your hair will grow back and there are newer drugs to minimize nausea. In contrast, if you decide that chemotherapy is not the optimal path for you, and your doctors agree, then embrace your decision and cast away lingering ambivalence. What is "right" for one person may not be "right" for you.

Update: Oncotype Testing

Since my diagnosis, Oncotype testing has expanded, becoming available to more candidates, including some women with lymph node involvement or DCIS. Ask your doctor for details. Read more about Oncotype testing at genomichealth.com.

A Picture Says at Least a Thousand Words

No way around it, hair loss *is* tough.

As a teenager in the 70s, inspired by "Charlie's Angels," I had Farrah-like, layered curls created with hot rollers. During the 80s, I went with huge, spiral-permed mall hair, styled daily with a diffuser. In the 90s, I mimicked Ivana Trump's lacquered bouffant, which required a copious amount of mousse.

My kids always have a good laugh anytime we bring out the old photo albums. They especially crack up over pictures of me in an acid-washed denim jumpsuit or neon leg warmers.

Everyone dreads the hair loss associated with chemo. I decide to be proactive and cut my shoulder-length tresses to ease the transition.

Liz and Hannah accompany me to the salon, where we thumb through glossy style magazines, looking for inspiration.

"I think you should get this one!" Hannah points to an asymmetrical punk-rock design.

"No, this is more me." I hold up a photo. "Check out the modified mohawk."

When Mandy, my hair stylist, calls me back to her station, I explain why I'm making such a drastic change.

"I'm so sorry," she says. "But don't worry; we'll get you a fun, sassy look."

I introduce her to Liz and Hannah, who sit nearby in empty client chairs.

"Could you turn me around? So I can talk with my friends?"

"Good idea!" she says, picking up the scissors. "Then when I'm done, you can face the mirror for your big reveal."

"Yeah, maybe it'll feel like a makeover show."

Mandy starts snipping. Hunks of hair fall to the floor. Swallowing a lump of sadness, I pick up a clipping from my black plastic apron.

When I was a bald baby, Mom scotch-taped a bow to my head so people would know I was a girl. But not since infancy have I ever had super-short hair—not even when the Mia Farrow "pixie" and the Dorothy Hamill "wedge" were *en vogue*.

Overhearing our conversation, a woman in a nearby chair starts reciting a litany of all the people she's known who've had cancer, who've been through chemo, *blah, blah, blah.*

I roll my eyes at Hannah and Liz.

Then she starts yakking about the people she knows who've died of the disease.

Just what I want to hear.

I cringe, wishing I could stick my fingers in my ears.

Seeing my panicked expression, Liz hijacks the conversation. "No worries. She's going to be around a long time. In fact, we're making plans for our Girls Getaway Weekend."

"Yes," chimes in Hannah, sending Loudmouth Stranger an icy glare. "Joanna, what do you think? Beach or mountains?"

I appreciate their refocusing the conversation. The experience reminds me of when, right before my due date for Alex, I went for a relaxing pedicure—wanting my toes to look cute in those metal stirrups. Unfortunately, the client in the next chair shared a graphic accounting of her tortuous birth experience that culminated with a broken tailbone. I was already petrified about my first delivery, so her story turbocharged my anxiety.

So much for my relaxing spa experience. They never seem to go as planned.

Finally, the stylist's scissors fall silent. "All done."

"Looks good!" Liz insists.

"Very nice," adds Hannah.

I brace myself as Mandy spins my chair around. Staring back from the mirror is a short-haired stranger.

~

For the rest of the day, I keep checking my reflection, perennially surprised. My hair has always been thick with a somewhat coarse texture, not silky like the tresses featured in the Clairol commercials. Though blonde as a child, my natural color has darkened to a light brown, and after my haircut, all the golden highlights are gone.

Frequently, when a woman gets one of those Hollywood makeovers, she looks vamped-up with a push-up bra and hair extensions. But in my situation, rather than having my feminine attributes enhanced, they're disappearing.

I wonder how I'll feel when my hair starts to fall out. *Will I lose all my hair or just some? Will I be self-conscious about my appearance? Will I look sickly?*

Dr. Point Guard has told me the chemotherapy regimen he's recommending might not cause complete hair loss. Some of his patients on this particular drug cocktail have only had thinning. But to me, having seen some women with a Donald Trump comb-over, sparse hair looks even worse than complete baldness. If I need to, I'll take charge and get my head shaved.

~

That night, when Ryan and the kids are asleep, I log onto the *YSC* message boards. One Pink Sister has posted a photo of the back of her bald head. Written across it in black marker are the words **THIS IS WHAT HEALING LOOKS LIKE**.

Wow.

Chills run down my spine. This picture doesn't say just a

thousand words. *More like a million!*

And the words. *Simple but powerful.*

What a paradigm shift, to see hair loss not as a sign of illness but as a symbol of strength and determination, a signal that the treatments are working, kicking cancer's ass and taking names. I won't be like Sampson, losing his strength once his long hair is cut. Instead, since I'm drowning in a sea of pink stuff anyway, I'll put on coordinating rose-colored glasses and change my perspective.

I stare at the photo, sending thankful vibes to the Pink Sister who posted it.

Yes, *this* is what healing looks like.

Divine Secret: Wear your baldness with pride; you are a pink warrior princess!

When you look in the mirror, hold your head high. Baldness is your metaphorical war paint, showing sinister, stealthy cancer you won't back down. I admire Pink Sisters who decorate their follicle-challenged scalps with gorgeous henna tattoos or wear "Bald is Beautiful" trucker hats. You rock!

♡ 31

Welcome to the Chemo-Spa

I've been procrastinating, reluctant to tell the kids about my impending chemo. To soften the news, I cook a roast with potatoes and carrots, one of my family's favorites. We chat about normal stuff over dinner, but when everyone's finished, I ask them to stay at the table.

"There's something we need to tell you," Ryan starts. He looks at me.

The kids freeze, worried there's more bad news.

"Everything's okay," I assure them. "I'm doing great. Just wanted to let you know I'll be starting chemotherapy soon."

"Chemo?" asks Alex, a shocked look on his face. "I thought your surgery got rid of the cancer."

"Chances are very good that it did," I explain. "The cancer's been evicted. Chemo's a precaution to make sure no squatter cells are left behind."

The boys slump in their chairs, puzzled.

"Look at it this way, guys. Sometimes bad cells can grow in your body, like weeds in a garden. Chemo is sort of like hosing them down with weed killer."

Not a bad analogy since chemo is toxic by definition.

"Are you going to lose your hair?" asks Nick.

"Maybe. Well, probably."

"Mommy's going to be bald?" pipes up Larissa, giggling.

Suddenly, I feel both relieved and exasperated. I'd been thinking about buying my daughter the "Chemo Kimmie" rag doll I'd seen in a magazine. Designed to help children cope with the anxiety of cancer, the hairless doll comes equipped with two wigs and a bandanna. But since my daughter views a bald Mommy as potentially funny—rather than traumatic—she may not need it.

Divine Secret: Check out resources to help your children understand what's happening.

The Kimmie Cares doll, available at kimmiecares.com, is a great product for kids, helping to lessen their anxiety over a loved one's appearance.

Nowhere Hair, a children's book written by Sue Glader and illustrated by Edith Buenen, explains cancer and the effects of treatment in a relatable and vibrant tone.

Camp Kesem is a weeklong sleepaway summer camp for children age 6 to 16 who have a parent with cancer. For more info, check out campkesem.org.

~

A few days later, I pause outside the Cancer Center entrance, trying to calm my jitters. Today is chemotherapy orientation, where I'll learn about side effects and precautions.

Chemo-Teach Nurse escorts me to a small conference room and hands me a folder. "Feeling okay? Ready to start chemo?"

"I'm nervous, but the sooner I start, the sooner I finish."

"That's a common feeling."

Chemo-Teach Nurse describes a typical treatment day. "After checking in, you'll go to the on-site lab for blood work. If the numbers look good, you'll be called back to the chemo cubicles. Then the nurse will start an IV line with saline solution."

Great, more needles.

"We want you hydrated. It's important to drink lots of fluids—preferably water—while undergoing treatment."

My bladder's the size of a thimble, so I hope my cubicle is next to the bathroom.

"We'll give you meds to alleviate nausea and help prevent allergic reaction."

I nod.

"In addition to the steroid medications you're taking by mouth, you'll receive more steroids via IV. Then we'll start the two chemo drugs your doctor has ordered."

"How long does a treatment session take?"

"It varies, but usually around six hours. Most people bring a friend or family member. You'll need someone to drive you home."

"My husband's coming."

"Good. Each patient area has a flat-screen TV and DVD player to help pass the time."

Chemo-Teach Nurse tells me about the chemo drugs I've been prescribed and their common side effects. I'm relieved to forego one drug nicknamed the "Red Devil" due to its potential to cause severe nausea and corrosive skin damage.

"Your oncologist has prescribed four treatments for you, three weeks apart, but keep in mind that timetables can change. Sometimes we have to push treatment back a week or two, depending on how your body responds."

Hope that doesn't happen. Three months is plenty long enough!

For at least the next twelve weeks, I'll be dealing with possible achy flu-like feelings, pain in my extremities and joints, low-grade fever, queasiness, headache, hair loss, nail damage, metallic taste, and constipation.

"A little low-grade fever is not unusual," Chemo-Teach Nurse explains. "But if your temperature reaches 100.5, call us immediately."

"Okay."

"Usually, you'll feel the worst several days after treatment. Then the side effects will start to subside."

She points to a chart in my information packet. "Remember, day five through day ten is when your blood counts are low and you are most susceptible to infection. Use plenty of hand sanitizer and stay away from people with colds, flu, or any contagious disease."

"No worries. I've got tons of hand sanitizer. Plus some surgical masks and latex gloves. Guess I went a little wacky over the bird flu scare."

"O…kay." Chemo-Teach Nurse seems uncertain what to say.

"Got a closet full of toilet paper and tuna fish, too. Let me know if you ever need some."

She gives me a perplexed look, but doesn't laugh. "How about I give you a tour of the infusion area?"

"Sure."

I follow her down the hall, away from patient exam rooms, past the reception desk, and through some double doors. There's a small waiting area on the right and a lab for blood draws on the left. As we walk into the treatment area, I notice a large aquarium filled with brightly-colored fish. Windows overlook a courtyard with shrubbery and a fountain.

Pretty fly place, I think, admiring the beige recliners. Each cubicle has a wood and frosted glass divider providing some privacy. With decorative lighting and flat screen TVs, it resembles an upscale beauty salon.

Yet the sarcastic voice in my head, echoing Vincent Price, grows louder.

Welcome to the Chemo-Spa!

(Cue audio effects of werewolf howls and the flapping wings of screeching bats.)

Today, instead of highlighting and styling your hair, we'll make it fall out. We won't manicure your nails, but we might make them turn black and

Divine Secret: Drink plenty of water so you'll be hydrated before lab draws and IVs.

With juicy, plumped-up veins and a skillful health care worker, the needle pricks can be as slight as a tiny bug bite. But if you're dehydrated, it can feel like somebody's digging into your flesh with a steak knife.

Divine Secret: Make your time at the Chemo-Spa as comfortable as possible.

Plan to wear comfy clothes and fluffy socks. Pack a bag with your own pillow, DVDs, or anything else to help you stay distracted and relaxed. Put together a playlist of motivational music.

Some suggested tracks:
- "Stronger" by Kelly Clarkson
- "I Run for Life" by Melissa Etheridge
- "It's Not My Time" by Three Doors Down
- "Stand" by Rascal Flatts
- "I'm Not Afraid" by Eminem
- "It's My Life" by Bon Jovi
- "Survivor" by Destiny's Child
- "Not Gonna Give Into It" by Olivia Newton John

crumble. Maybe you'll lose weight from nausea or gain weight from the steroids. Who knows? As a bonus, after several appointments, you'll receive a complimentary Brazilian bikini wax!

Bwah, ha, ha!

Is it too late to change my reservation to the Canyon Ranch?

Walking the length of the room, I smile at the volunteers handing out blankets, magazines, and snacks. But seeing the actual patients is a bit anticlimactic. Many are watching TV; some are napping. They appear tired, but not outwardly tortured or terrified. If they can get through this, I can, too.

♡ 32

Greetings, Chemo-Sabe!

Today's my first chemo session. I'm scheduled to have four rounds of treatment, scheduled every three weeks. The number of treatments and length of time between them will differ for each patient, based on the patient's circumstances. Some people undergo what's called "dose-dense" treatment every two weeks. Ladies with a subtype of breast cancer called Her/2 positive are usually advised to schedule a weekly infusion of the drug Herception for a year.

Originally, I'd planned on asking one of my funniest friends—maybe Liz or Justine—to accompany me because they'd make snarky jokes instead of acting saccharine sweet. However, Ryan insists he wants to go, which I appreciate, even though he won't be a barrel of fun.

As Chemo-Teach Nurse explained, after a blood draw I'm escorted to the infusion area. It's a busy day; almost all the cubicles are occupied. I walk past fellow patients, some of whom appear to be in robust health, others looking frail, curled up beneath blankets, scarves or hats covering their heads.

How will I feel after several rounds of chemo? Will makeup and a cute wig help me blend in, like the models from the "Look Good, Feel Better" workshop? Or will my appearance scream Cancer Patient?

I hear muffled TV sounds and watch nurses flit back and forth, tending to the obnoxious warning beeps of medical equipment.

Bubbly Nurse Navigator, wearing a pink cowgirl hat and carrying pom-poms, comes over to my cubicle to say hello. She works with Dr. Point Guard and the other oncologists at this location, helping patients manage all aspects of their treatment. Even though I had my mastectomy performed at a different hospital, Bubbly Nurse Navigator mailed me a pre-surgical care package with a soft camisole, small pillow, and other helpful items.

"How are you today?" she asks. "Ready for your first treatment?"

"Ready as I'll ever be."

"Let me give you the official welcome." She shakes her pom-poms and does a little cheer: *"New chemo patient, you're a pearl! Now take your drugs so you don't hurl!"*

While I laugh, Ryan looks slightly embarrassed.

I settle into my recliner. Infusion Nurse taps my left wrist and hand, searching for a good vein. She ties a strap of stretchy rubber around my arm and plunges in the needle. *Ouch!* After starting a saline drip, she leaves to check on other patients.

Minutes later, Cheerful Volunteer, a gray-haired woman wearing a hospital auxiliary vest, stops by to chat. "Would you like a blanket?"

"I'd love one, thanks." The room is surprisingly chilly, so the warm fabric feels good spread across my lap.

"How about a snack? Something to drink?"

"A ginger ale, please."

She brings me a big Styrofoam cup filled with ice and soda.

"I've been where you are, dear," she says, patting my shoulder. "Let me know if you need anything."

"Thank you."

As she walks away, I'm thinking how nice it is that she comes to offer support and comfort. I'm also thinking those Oreos on her cart look pretty good. Will have to keep them in mind for later.

I turn on the TV and surf the channels. Talk shows, soap operas, dated sitcoms, infomercials. *How can there be so many TV stations but nothing good to watch?*

I flip past a cable news channel.

"Hey, go back one."

Drats! Now I'll be listening to an endless loop of news stories. Ryan obsesses at times over Fox News. I suspect he's crushing on the gorgeous anchorwomen wearing gallons of shiny lip gloss, apparently mandated by their TV contracts.

"Here." I hand him the remote.

If I'd brought Mom or a girlfriend, we'd be watching a funny chick flick. But my husband's here out of love, so I should act appreciative, not annoyed.

I retrieve a magazine from my chemo supply bag. I'll read.

These infusions take time. I don't have any reaction to the saline solution—other than having to wheel my IV pole into the restroom—but after Infusion Nurse adds Benadryl, I feel drowsy. I recline my chair and lift the footrest. Ryan turns on his laptop while I doze.

When I wake up, it's almost noon.

"Are you hungry?" Ryan asks. "I can get something from the cafeteria."

"Sounds good."

"Any requests?"

"Surprise me."

~

About ten minutes later, Ryan returns with two plates of the daily special: roasted chicken, rice, and green beans. We're eating and watching a PBS documentary when Cheerful Volunteer stops by. "Would you like some sandwiches? I have roast beef, turkey, or tuna salad."

My mouth full of chicken, I shake my head "No."

"Oh, well. I see you have something already. That looks good, too."

I can read Ryan's mind. He's wishing he'd known about the *perfectly good, free sandwiches* before spending money at the cafeteria.

Before he can comment, my IV machine starts beeping, indicating that the plastic drip is empty. Infusion Nurse wheels over her cart of medical supplies.

"I'm going to start your first chemotherapeutic agent now," she says, detaching the empty plastic bag and tethering another one. "This may cause a strong flushing sensation. Let me know if this happens, and I'll give you more Benadryl."

This is the moment the toxins first flood my bloodstream. There's something very counterintuitive about choosing to pump your body full of poison to rid it of disease. I wish we could destroy the evil, malignant cells without punishing the nice, well-behaved ones.

At first, I feel nothing…then my chest and throat tighten. A strange warmth surges through my veins. Every inch of my body fills with hot liquid, as if my IV line is hooked up to a Starbucks espresso machine.

More than any previous time in my life, I'm so aware of the dichotomy between body and mind, I can't help feeling rattled by this weird physical reaction that is out of my control. The fact that I inhabit a temporal house of flesh and bone comes into sharp focus. My spirit is strong, but my body is fragile.

I press the call button.

By the time Infusion Nurse arrives, the sensation is subsiding.

"You're a little flushed," she says, attaching another bag to the IV pole. "This is not uncommon. I'm going to slow down your drip and give you more Benadryl."

Divine Secret: Choose a compatible chemo-buddy, if possible.

Ask someone who will be supportive in the way that you need. As for me, I wouldn't want someone who'd act overly sad, serious, and sympathetic to the point where I'd be comforting them. Despite getting annoyed with him at times, I'm glad my husband went with me. It meant a lot to have him there.

Okay, enough drama for today! I could use a few therapeutic Oreos, so I flag down Cheerful Volunteer.

~

After another catnap, I awaken when Infusion Nurse returns to start my second chemo drip.

"You probably won't have any immediate reaction to this drug like you did with the last, but it'll catch up with you. Within a day or two, you may feel flu-like symptoms, achiness, low-grade fever, fatigue."

"Not nausea?"

"Not as bad with this drug as some others. Still, you may feel queasy, so make sure to stay on top of it. Keep taking the oral nausea meds your oncologist prescribed."

I glare at my newest bag of poison, as if it can be cowed by my intimidating stare. Hey, chemo, I threw up all during the first trimesters of two pregnancies, so I know my way around a barf bag! I'm not scared! You're not the boss of me!

Meanwhile, my insides quiver like that bowl of green hospital jello.

~

By late afternoon, my last infusion complete, I'm released to go home. When we hear a cheerful commotion, I look down the aisle and see Bubbly Nurse Navigator, once again donning her pink cowgirl hat. She's waving pom-poms, shouting a cheer to celebrate someone's final treatment. A volunteer is cutting slices of a vanilla cake with pink decorative frosting.

On our way out, we offer congratulations to the happy patient.

"Would you like some?" Bubbly Nurse Navigator holds up a plate.

"Not today." I'm ready to go home. "I'll look forward to my own chemo farewell party!"

She smiles. "Take it day by day. It'll be here before you know it."

~

As we walk to the parking lot, Ryan holds my hand. I squeeze back, glancing at the plastic hospital bracelet encircling my wrist.

"Thanks for coming with me today, honey."

"Of course! I wanted to be here with you."

"I really appreciate it."

"But next time, we're gonna wait for the free sandwiches."

I laugh out loud.

Fighting Germs and Stupidity

R esting at home for the first few days after chemo, I update my blog and check e-mail. The encouraging messages swaddle me in a cloud of love. My *CaringBridge* account keeps everyone updated without me answering a zillion questions. Friends and family can compose and edit their thoughts instead of blurting out words on the spot. Most people mean well, even if they make awkward comments such as, "Oh, my aunt died of breast cancer."

Thanks for sharing! That makes my day!

But I laugh when Cassidy, a kindergartner with the sweet face of a cherub and the outsized personality of a midget Bette Midler, shares a warning as we walk home from the school bus stop.

"Hey, Larissa's Mom!" Cassidy shouts. "I heard you have cancer."

"Yes, that's true."

She shakes her head in dismay, causing the enormous purple barrette that coordinates with her Gymboree dress to slide out of place. "Uh, I hate to tell you this," she says, a solemn expression on her face. "Cancer is very bad. It can kill you!"

"Yeah, so I've heard," I put my arm around Larissa. "Don't worry. I'm sticking around."

Cassidy's mother looks mortified, but I'm amused by the precocious comments.

I don't laugh though, a few hours later, when one of Larissa's friends rings the doorbell. Immediately I notice her Rudolph-red nose and hacking cough.

"Can Larissa play?" she asks.

"Aren't you sick, sweetie?"

"Yeah, but I took some medicine."

"Sorry," I tell her. "Larissa would love to play, but I can't be around anyone with a cold or the flu. Maybe you can come over later in the week."

Seeing the crushed look on her face, I feel guilty, even though I'm following medical advice to protect my weakened immune system.

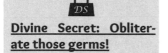

Divine Secret: Obliterate those germs!

If you're around snot-nosed—albeit adorable—young children, make sure you have disposable gloves, masks, Lysol, etc. on hand. (Those bird flu supplies came in handy after all!) Gently remind their playmates not to come over if contagious.

~

It's tough for friends and family to gauge my moods and calibrate their comments. I hate it when someone gives me a sad-eyed, hang-dog expression, as if my situation is pitiful. Yet at other times, I'm annoyed by people lamenting their kid not winning the spelling bee or making the travel soccer team, as if it's a family tragedy. Humor's my favorite coping mechanism, but other people's punch lines sound clumsy or obnoxious. *(Hint: if you're in the Pink Sorority, you're allowed to joke about getting perky new foobs. But if you're not in the club, don't go there!)*

Some people avoid me because talking about cancer makes them uncomfortable. I'd rather hear a stupid—though well-meaning—remark than feel they're dodging me. But please, spare me platitudes about God having a plan or purpose. Cancer isn't an Old Testament–style locust plague. Lousy, random stuff happens. I don't believe God is smacking my knuckles with His celestial ruler.

And while some people avoid mentioning the word "cancer" around me, others overstep their bounds, such as the bone-headed acquaintance who asks me, point blank, "Did they get it all? What's your prognosis?" Stunned by the intimacy of his question and not wanting to share personal details, I mumble something about good survival rates for early-stage breast cancer.

Although I didn't want to join this sorority, I'm grateful for the support and camaraderie it's offered me. I hate it when a Pink Sister is hurt by an insensitive comment, whether made by family, friends, colleagues, medical personnel, or strangers. For my own sanity, I decide to print up metaphorical "Stupid Passes" and pretend I'm handing them out like flags at a political rally. Not because these idiots *deserve* a pass, but because I don't want to waste time and energy fretting over careless remarks. Instead, I pledge to overlook the clumsy words and hear their intent.

Pink Sisters are often surprised by the reactions of others. Some people, especially those who have weathered a health crisis or serious loss, will reach out with an unbelievable generosity of spirit and understanding. These folks step up right away and seem to understand exactly what you need. Yet others will drift away, too uneasy and uncomfortable to be there for you. So, I vow to cherish the deepening of unexpected friendships and to remember that if certain people stay away, it's probably due to their own fears and anxieties, not a lack of feelings for me.

Divine Secret: Give everyone a Stupid Pass.

Don't waste your energy being upset over thoughtless comments. Imagine you're Oprah on her famous car-giveaway show. Point and shout, "You get a Stupid Pass! You get a Stupid Pass! Everyone gets a Stupid Pass!"

> **Resource:**
>
> *Help Me Live: 20 Things People with Cancer Want You to Know*, by Lori Hope. This book helps bridge the communication gap between those waging a personal war against cancer and the "civilians" in their lives.

Over the next few days, Infusion Nurse's warning about unpleasant side effects proves true; my bones become achy, my stomach queasy. Nothing appeals, but I manage to sip hot tea and nibble some toast. Food has a strange metallic flavor. Unpleasant smells intensify. Mostly, I'm exhausted and feverish. Though I feel lousy, my first chemotherapy treatment has not been as difficult as I'd imagined.

But the plot thickens when Larissa comes into our bedroom. "Mommy, I don't feel good." Her face is flushed, her forehead hot.

I fetch the thermometer. Her fever has spiked to 101.3.

Yikes! What do I do?

Sick children want to cuddle with their mommies, but my immune system is seriously compromised. A run-of-the-mill cold could hospitalize me, which would complicate life for everyone.

After giving Larissa ibuprofen and a glass of water, I settle her on the couch with a pillow and her favorite blanket. I turn on a PBS kids show, wash my hands, and call Mom. She'd driven home a few days ago, since I was managing okay. I'm sure she's tired of sleeping in Alex's cluttered room, surrounded by rocket ship models and Pinewood Derby trophies.

"Sorry to be calling in the cavalry so soon. You didn't even have time to unpack."

"What's wrong?"

I fill her in on Larissa's symptoms.

"You shouldn't be around her if she's running a fever. I'll come to your house. You need to pack a bag and stay here with Pop for a few days."

I'm leery of turning into a crazed germophobe like Howard Hughes, isolated in a room full of tissues and bleach. However, chemo dangerously suppresses your body's ability to ward off infection, so I can't ignore the risk.

I wonder: *what do single moms do in this situation?* How tough it must be when you're the only adult, knowing that if you get too close to a sick child, you could jeopardize your own health and need hospitalization. You can't send a child with an illness to school or daycare. Many babysitters won't care for a child with a contagious illness. I feel so bad for my Pink Sisters who don't have family or friends willing to pitch in.

Within hours, Mom shows up. I leave to spend a few germ-free days in the mountains with Pop. While she's dealing with cranky kids, homework, and laundry, I'm sitting on the front porch talking, reading, and watching the sunset.

I admit this is a sweet deal; I might be tempted to stick Larissa's thermometer in the toaster oven sometime!

Divine Secret: Fear is often worse than reality.

My neurotic imagination runs wild at times, expecting the worst. No one would name me a poster girl for excellent mental health. Take it one day, one hour, one minute at a time.

Copy and clip as needed:

Stupid Pass

Name:_____

Date:_____

Comment:_____

_____

Stupid Pass

Name:_____

Date:_____

Comment:_____

_____

Stupid Pass

Name:_____

Date:_____

Comment:_____

_____

Hair Today, Gone Tomorrow

October 2007

Once Larissa's fever passes, I return home.

Thanks to Tessa, someone delivers a home-cooked meal every night, which has turned into a real boon for Ryan and the kids. Tonight we have a chicken casserole with salsa, rice, black beans, and tortilla chips.

"I'd give the Mexican chicken five stars," says Ryan.

"Me, too," says Alex. "Can you ask for the recipe?"

"Yeah, I like this," adds Nick. "But the lemony baked fish? Don't get that recipe!"

"Who made you guys food critics?"

Almost every meal receives four or five stars, setting the culinary bar way too high for me.

Unfortunately, I can't personally appreciate all the wonderful meals since chemo has taken away my appetite. The inside of my mouth feels sandpapery. Nothing tastes like it should. My queasiness wanes, but the achiness continues.

Divine Secret: Chemo is not the time for calorie counting.

Milkshakes for breakfast, lunch, and dinner? Why not, if it sounds appealing? Now available in a variety of delicious flavors: chocolate, cardboard, or stainless steel.

I've heard that hair loss usually begins about two weeks after your first chemo treatment, so I'm not surprised when mine collects like a bird's nest in the shower drain.

The lightest touch causes strands to fall away. I stand at the mirror transfixed and horrified.

I expected this. I prepared for this, but…

It's like a kick in my stomach, making me feel vulnerable. I remind myself of the "THIS IS WHAT HEALING LOOKS LIKE" photograph. But I'm not feeling much like a warrior princess at the moment.

When the doorbell rings, I tear myself away from the strange reflection.

Liz is on the doorstep, holding out a vanilla latte. "You look good. Feeling okay?"

"Not too bad."

"Losing any hair yet?"

I gently tug a hunk of hair. It falls away in a large clump.

Liz jumps, visibly startled. "That's an image imprinted in my brain."

"Didn't mean to scare you." I laugh, mainly because I don't want to cry. "Guess I'll have that Kojak look before long."

Divine Secret: Join the Sisterhood of the Traveling Pants— PINK VERSION.

Check out hopescarves.org, an organization that allows women to send their freshly cleaned, previously worn scarves to women experiencing hair loss due to cancer, injury, or illness, along with a personal note of support.

Waking up the following morning, I find my pillowcase covered with loose strands. I remember that Hospital Beautician, who taught the "Look Good, Feel Better" class, offered to shave my head when needed, something she does for lots of patients. It's time for an appointment.

I dread getting my head shaved, but watching it fall out is worse.

Grabbing my purse and keys, I stop at the door. I don't need to do this alone.

Picking up the phone, I call Justine, whose sensitive heart lurks beneath her smart-alecky sense of humor. "Do you have plans this morning?" I ask.

"No, I'm free. What's up?"

"Okay," I take a deep breath. "I hate to ask you—or anyone—to do this, but my hair is falling out. Please don't feel obligated, but I was hoping you'd go to the salon with me."

"Of course I'll go. I'll pick you up in ten minutes."

"Thanks, Justine!"

"How about we have lunch after your appointment? Then stop by the mall for an hour or two?"

"That sounds great!" Justine is a true believer in retail therapy. Her knack for finding terrific bargains makes her one of my favorite shopping companions. Today's not our usual jaunt to the mall, but her presence will make things easier.

~

At the Cancer Care Center, Hospital Beautician greets us and directs me to a chair. "Did you bring your wig?"

"Yes."

"Good, I'll trim it for you." Wrapping a plastic poncho around my shoulders, she gives me a reassuring pat. "I know this is hard, but it's temporary. Your hair will grow back."

I watch in the mirror as Hospital Beautician runs the razor along my scalp.

At this moment, the cancer is real. So scary and ugly.

It will grow back, it will grow back, it will grow back...

"Can you make me resemble Demi Moore in *G.I. Jane*?" I ask, attempting a feeble joke.

"The bald look worked for her," adds Justine.

"I'll do my best."

"I'll settle for a young Sinead O'Conner. Just don't make me look like Yul Brynner or Elmer Fudd."

I force a smile and exchange glances with Justine. I see tears welling in her eyes. My eyes are teary too, but I blink them away. It takes only a few minutes before my head is completely shorn. It's jarring to confront this bald stranger in the mirror, so I repeat the mantra in my head: *this is what healing looks like, this is what healing looks like...*

I'm not sure why I want to document the occasion, but I hand Justine my cell phone and ask her to take a photo. Bald is definitely not a great look for me.

Hospital Beautician brushes the clippings from my shoulders and helps me put on my wig. It's too big and puffy—even for a native Texan like me—so she trims the bangs and sides.

"Now this is one cute wig!" she declares.

"It looks good, Jo," Justine adds.

Looking in the mirror, I feel self-conscious. *Is it obvious I'm wearing a wig? Or could this pass as my natural hair if someone didn't know better?* I'll admit it's shinier and bouncier than my own hair, so that's a plus.

"Let's have some lunch," Justine suggests. "Then we can shop for some headbands to change up your new look."

As we dine at the restaurant and walk through the mall, I continue feeling self-conscious, like I'm wearing a halo of neon lights rather than an artificial hairpiece.

Nevertheless, lunch and shopping with a friend make a lousy day a little bit better.

> **Divine Secret: Don't be too proud to ask for support.**
>
> I could have gone to the salon by myself, but it was easier having a friend along to boost my courage. You don't have to face sad, scary experiences alone.

~

On Sunday morning, I'm feeling good enough to attend church. We're greeted warmly by other parishioners, who've been generous in bringing meals and sending cards.

Yet along with the prayers, I'm getting stares. People are trying their best not to zero in on my bust line, even making intense eye contact with me to avoid gazing downward. But to be human is to be curious. Everyone tries to be discreet, but many can't prevent themselves from taking covert glances.

I feel self-conscious and awkward, like I'm the overturned 18-wheeler and they're the motorists who can't stop rubber-necking.

After Sunday school, we settle into a pew in the sanctuary. Crazy Uncle Harry takes the podium to make some announcements.

"Ya'll come out this Thursday night for the square dance. We'll have snacks and a professional caller," he says. "Besides, fellas, let me tell you something. Your wife's gonna look a whole lot sexier when she's dancing!"

The congregation erupts into laughter. Crazy Uncle Harry's wife turns as scarlet as the dress she's wearing. Guess I'm not the only one feeling embarrassed today.

During the service, Barry leads the congregation in prayer. He asks God for healing and strength for several church members undergoing chemo-therapy—namely, an older man battling leukemia and me. As several hundred people bow their heads in accordance, lifting us up in concern, I feel buoyant, like I'm the subject of the jokey bumper sticker *God Loves You. But I'm His Favorite!*

There's such power knowing that—*at this exact moment*—all these people hold me in their hearts, wishing me healing and comfort.

Divine Secret: It's not your imagination. People are staring at your body like it's a billboard.

Call it intrusive and rude or awkward and embarrassing. Friends, neighbors, and colleagues will try not to look, but the urge will be impossible to resist. So just accept it. Don't let it unnerve you. I felt self-conscious wearing my wig and my clone in public for the first few times, but I couldn't have revealed my new "style" in a more supportive place.

Pinktober—My Least Favorite Month

October used to be my favorite month. Every year, I looked forward to seeing the gold and crimson leaves, watching college football, and handing out Halloween candy to neighborhood ninjas and princesses.

I still enjoy the cool, crisp days. But now October has morphed into "Pinktober," a month many survivors secretly dread. After experiencing surgery, chemotherapy, and hair loss, I've had more than enough awareness, thank you very much!

Don't get me wrong—breast cancer awareness is a good thing. Many survivors embrace the deluge of pink, donning shirts, hats, jewelry—anything to get people to learn more about the disease, get a mammogram, or donate to support research and treatment. Numerous corporations and individuals give generously, but many others jump on the marketing bandwagon, making negligible contributions. And when a company slaps a pink ribbon on a product containing known carcinogens, you can bet that a posse of Pink Sisters notice.

Going to the grocery store generates sensory overload, a bombardment in every aisle. I'm surrounded by pink ribbons plastered on soup cans, toilet paper packaging, yogurt cartons...

Yet, I'm touched by the pretty pink jewelry I've received, even if I don't want to be a walking, sparkling advertisement. One of my artistic aunts made me a stunning glass and metal pendant that always inspires compliments. A friend gave me a glittery hot pink rhinestone pin that brings on the bling. I love the inspirational silver bracelets, comfy pink pajamas, and hand-knitted shawls people have sent.

Divine Secret: Beware of "Pink-Washing."

Some corporations will use pink ribbon imagery to market their products—including some that contain known or suspected carcinogens—but donate little to no portion of the proceeds to breast cancer research. Calling for transparency and account-ability, Breast Cancer Action (bcaction.org) developed the Think Before You Pink cam-paign.

But I confess that I'm not crazy about the breast aware-ness calendar featuring black and white portraits of sur-vivors. Miss January is bald, scarred, and topless. As is Miss February, Miss March, Miss April, etc. I appreciate the sender's good intentions, but if I want to view a bald, scarred woman, I can just check the mirror.

~

Overwhelmed by a deluge of pinkness and feeling the claustro-phobia of cabin fever, I attend a meeting of the downtown sup-port group, where we assemble gift bags for an upcoming fund-raiser. I cover my bald head with a brown felt fedora because, if there's any place I should feel okay about my appearance, it's around Pink Sisters. My wig is fairly cute, but wearing it for too long at a time gives me a tension headache.

Over wine and pizza, I quiz the women on their treatment and reconstruction choices.

"I wanted to do chemo!" Floral Hat Girl insists. "I kept telling myself I'm too young for this, so I insisted on a double mastec-tomy. My breasts seemed like the enemy. I couldn't trust them anymore. I have a strong family history, even though none of us have tested positive for any known BRCA gene pre-disposi-tions."

"My surgeon said I didn't need chemo," counters Curvy Italian Lady. "So I had a lumpectomy and radiation. No puking or hair loss for me! But radiation was exhausting. Nobody warned me!"

Statuesque Red-Head pours herself a refill of chardonnay. "Yeah, and nobody warned me about the chance of permanent skin damage from radiation. My chest looks like a burned taquito from 7-11."

We all laugh, because sometimes that's the only thing you can do.

Everyone seems willing to share, so I ask, "Did any of you have immediate reconstruction?"

"I had expanders put in during my double mastectomy," Floral Hat Girl says, reaching for another slice of pizza. "But there's nothing immediate about it. It's a process. Now that they've been swapped I'm reasonably happy. Glad to be done."

"Let me share one piece of advice," adds Statuesque Red-Head. "Make sure you talk to more than one plastic surgeon. Most doctors either specialize in, or prefer, one method and that's where they will steer you. Make sure you learn about all your options."

"I had expanders put in during my bilateral, too," says Petite Blonde, shaking her head. "But it's been a nightmare! They found positive lymph nodes." Reaching into her pocket, she pulls out a tissue. "It's been three months and I'm still having healing issues. I can't start chemo yet."

"Oh, sweetie, we're so sorry." Curvy Italian Lady gives her a hug.

"You hang in there," adds Silky Scarf Chick, patting her shoulder. "Call us anytime you need to talk."

We all add murmurs of empathy and support.

"We need chocolate!" Statuesque Red-Head picks up a plate of brownies. "Anybody want one?"

"Heck, yeah," declares Silky Scarf Chick. "I don't care if they're organic or not!"

Curvy Italian Lady chooses a brownie, then stops with it

midway to her mouth. She turns toward Silky Scarf Chick. "Didn't you get a DIEP reconstruction recently?"

"Yes, a couple of months ago. I had to go to New Orleans. And I'm so glad I did! I hated the idea of an implant. Didn't want a foreign object in my body."

Divine Secret: Graciously accept the offer of a "Show and Tell."

I regret that my embarrassment stopped a Pink Sister from unveiling her recent DIEP reconstruction. Her willingness to share was generous and brave; my stupid prudishness may have come across as unkind and ungrateful.

"Did you have a single or bilateral?" I ask.

"Single. Just the cancer side. I wanted to keep my remaining natural breast."

All eyes focus on Silky Scarf Chick's blouse, but since we're at a Ta-Ta sorority meeting, this isn't a breach of etiquette.

"Wow, nice job," says Floral Hat Girl.

"Yeah, I got good symmetry." She starts unbuttoning her shirt. "Would you like to see?"

"Uh, that's okay," I stammer, my face as red as the pepperoni slices on the pizza. "But thanks for offering. You look fabulous."

"Yes, girlfriend. You look mah-ve-lous!" Statuesque Red-Head raises her wineglass. "To foobs!"

We clink together in a toast. Sometimes wine and chocolate—in moderation, of course—are just what the doctor ordered.

Update: More surgical options are available today.

When I was diagnosed in 2007, only a handful of surgeons were qualified to perform DIEP. Now, chances are you'll find an in-state surgeon trained in microsurgical reconstruction techniques. Check out all your options, weighing them by your own personal rubric.

36

Statistically Speaking

Since I know what to expect, my second trip to the Chemo-Spa is less unnerving. After unpacking a book, several magazines, and a DVD, I settle into the recliner. A nurse starts my IV. A volunteer offers drinks and snacks.

After they walk away, Ryan looks up from his laptop. "That reminds me. I'm not going to the cafeteria. Today we wait for the free sandwiches!"

"Okay, okay, Prince Cheapskate—uh, I mean Prince Charming."

The infusion room isn't as crowded this time, yet there are plenty of patients bundled beneath blankets, waiting for toxins to course through their veins. Sitting in my chemotherapy cubicle, I don't feel much like a fighter, or even an active participant. Despite the war imagery, my role feels somewhat passive, as if I'm the battlefield where opposing forces skirmish, inevitably scarred by collateral damage, no matter which side prevails.

After watching a forgettable comedy, I drift off to sleep, drowsy from the Benadryl drip. Ryan nudges me awake when a volunteer passes out ham and turkey sandwiches.

"Mind if I watch the news?"

I roll my eyes. With their sexy hair extensions and fake eyelashes, these glamorous Fox News chicks are getting on my nerves. Nevertheless, I hand him the remote.

"Pretty good sandwiches, huh?"

"Delicious," I reply, laying on sarcasm as thick as the mustard. I've heard women on diets say "nothing tastes as good as *thin*." Ryan's motto is "nothing tastes as good as *free*."

Infusion Nurse returns to begin my first chemo drug. Once again, after a few minutes, an unsettling wave of warmth crescendos inside me. My chest feels tight, so I press the call button.

Infusion Nurse races to my cubicle, then hooks me up to an oxygen mask. She pages a nurse practitioner. All this attention—though reassuringly prompt and thorough—makes me nervous. At my first treatment, if the nurses had swarmed me like this, I'd have panicked.

"I'm giving you more steroids," Infusion Nurse explains. "And I'm slowing down the chemo drip to reduce the flushing sensation."

The nurse practitioner listens to my heart and pronounces everything normal. After a few minutes on the dialed-down dosage, the warm tingling recedes.

By late afternoon, my body's been pumped with a second chemo agent, so I'm released to go home. I walk through the parking lot, tired and drained, but not miserable, relieved to have completed another treatment session.

~

Over the next few days, I fend off another round of nausea, achy flu-like feelings, and low-grade fever. But according to the information folder Chemo-Teach Nurse gave me, my side effects are typical.

Happy to be done with my second treatment, Ryan and I go to Larissa's Saturday afternoon soccer game. It's unseasonably hot, so instead of wearing my wig, I put on a fringe of "hat hair," a lightweight halo of tresses designed to give the illusion of hair under a baseball cap.

Later that evening, the boys have plans with friends, so we take Larissa to one of our favorite Italian restaurants. I bring my own plastic silverware to minimize the persistent metallic flavor. Despite some residual queasiness, the pasta with red sauce and fresh mozzarella is delicious, unlike most meals lately.

After Larissa goes to bed, Ryan and I watch a DVD. He pops popcorn and I add a few Milk Duds to my bowl for a sweet and salty treat. During the movie, I start feeling twinges of pain in my mid-section. We go to bed, but I don't sleep well.

~

Divine Secret: Eat tummy-friendly chemo snacks.

I avoided undercooked meat, unpasteurized cheeses, raw vegetables. Washed my hands constantly. But I'm no Einstein. The crunchy, gooey combo of popcorn and caramel? I should have just dipped steel wool sponges into a vat of chocolate fondue and eaten that!

I continue to hurt on Sunday. The crampy feeling doesn't subside, despite a warm bath and ibuprofen. I check the information folder again, but my temperature's not elevated enough for concern. Maybe it's constipation, a common chemo side effect. Or even something unrelated to cancer, such as bad premenstrual cramps.

Not wanting to disturb Ryan's sleep Sunday night, I stay downstairs on the sofa, dozing off during late-night cable shows, only to awake minutes later as the pain rouses me.

First thing Monday morning I call Chemo-Teach Nurse, but she isn't unduly worried. My treatment follow-up appointment is scheduled with Dr. Point Guard the next day. Besides, with a long history of wicked migraines, this pain isn't the worst I've endured. I decide to muddle through the next 24 hours. Ryan offers to stay home, but I insist he go to the office. *I'll be fine.*

Once everyone leaves for school or work, the house is silent.

I curl up on the bed, trying to ignore the vise squeezing my insides. Exhausted, I dissolve into the sensation, focusing all attention inward, like a woman in labor. Everything starts to fade, the edges of my surroundings becoming blurry. I withdraw into the pain, deep beneath flesh and muscle and bone, becoming less and less present, like a miniscule roly-poly coiled in a defensive ball. I flicker, my mind blank and static-y.

I glance at the clock. *Midafternoon?* I've spent the day curled in a fetal position on the bed, lacking the energy or desire to eat or drink, not even a cup of tea. Hours have passed while I've drifted along, unaware.

Suddenly, it's not the pain that's scaring me; it's the hazy sense of dissolving. Something's wrong.

I need rest. I'll close my eyes and hope the pain subsides.

I vacillate on what to do.

I'm so...so...tired.

An instinct deep inside commands me to gather every crumb of willpower and pick up the phone.

First, I call a neighbor, asking her to get Larissa from the bus stop. Then, I call Chemo-Teach Nurse. "Sorry to bother you again, but can anyone see me today?"

"I'll see what I can do. You don't want to wait until tomorrow, for the appointment with your regular oncologist?"

"No. If you can't work me in, I'm going to the emergency room."

"Okay," she says. "How soon can you be here?"

I get dressed and call Ryan to come home.

Divine Secrets: Heed the internal voice.

Pay attention when you have a feeling that something is wrong. Listen to your body and heed its warnings.

~

We check into the Cancer Center. Minutes later, I'm called back to an exam room and asked to describe my symptoms. I still don't have much fever, but when the nurse practitioner presses on my abdomen, I wince.

"You look a bit swollen, so to be safe, I'm sending you for a CT scan."

"Thank you," I mumble.

A burly orderly shows up with a gurney, which I ride like a magic carpet to the radiology department. Instead of cooling my heels in the waiting room with a beeper—like regular folk—my cancer VIP status upgrades me to a private waiting area. But rather than champagne and canapés, I'm given a large cup of vile-tasting barium suspension.

My stomach hurts. I'm sleep-deprived and have no appetite. I try to pretend I'm drinking a yummy peach Chik-Fil-A milkshake, but my taste buds recoil with every sip.

Please make it stop hurting!

Gray-Haired Taciturn Nurse keeps checking on me, insisting I finish the disgusting beverage. Making the experience even more unpleasant, she starts an IV. She has scant needle finesse, so the pain in my arm distracts me from the pain in my abdomen—somewhat like a primitive form of acupuncture.

With a final, frazzled surge of determination, I down the remaining liquid. I'm wheeled into the room with the CT scan and instructed to hold still as the machine hums, beeps, and thumps.

When the test is finished, I give the technician a weak smile. I point to my IV line. "Can you take this out?"

"Let's hold off until we hear from your doctor. We're paging him right now. As soon as we speak to him, we'll give you the phone."

Sigh. I close my eyes, hoping for pain relief soon.

In a few minutes, Dr. Point Guard is on the phone. "You must have had a little bird on your shoulder, telling you to come in."

"I don't know about that."

"Well, we need to admit you. The scan shows tiny perforations in your intestines. We're going to put you on strong antibiotics and hope things settle down."

"Okay."

"It's possible you'll need emergency surgery, but we're going to do our best to avoid that."

Emergency surgery? I feel a twinge of fear, but it's drowned out by pain and my bone-tired exhaustion.

"Your immune system is compromised by chemo," he continues, his voice serious yet reassuring. "We want to keep you out of the operating room if at all possible."

"Okay." I know he's telling me something important, but it doesn't sink in.

"A team of surgeons will keep close tabs on your status, and I'll be over to see you soon."

"May I make a quick trip home to pack a bag?"

"Absolutely not!" His pleasant voice takes on a stern tone. "You do not pass Go. You go directly to the oncology ward."

I'm puzzled by how this is unfolding. It never crossed my mind that I'd be admitted to the hospital. As an orderly wheels me to the elevator, I ask Ryan to go home and check on the kids, fix their dinner, and oversee homework—and to gather my toiletries, underwear, and slippers in an overnight bag. I should call Mom, but I tell myself I'll wait until morning. No point in making her worry.

As soon as I arrive in the oncology ward, surgeons traipse into my room, opening my flimsy cotton gown and scowling at my abdomen.

Dr. Point Guard walks in, a harried expression on his face. "You weren't supposed to end up here," he says. "But we're going to take good care of you."

"I know," I answer, tired and anxious. "Could I have something for the pain? And to help me sleep?"

"Certainly. I'll put in an order right now."

"Thanks."

"We need to let your digestive system calm down, so no eating or drinking for the next few days."

"Okay," I mumble.

After a while, the buzz of doctors and nurses subsides. While waiting for the medications to take effect, I remember a phrase

Dr. Point Guard often tells his patients: "You are an individual, not a statistic."

I think he says this to encourage patients who feel disheartened as they look at scary survival statistics. However, no matter the odds, someone falls on the losing end. At age 45, statistics said I probably wouldn't be diagnosed with cancer, but I lost that bet. Statistics said chemotherapy had a two to three percent chance of triggering heart failure or other serious side effect. I never expected to end up here, hospitalized for treatment complications. *Unlucky me, defying the odds yet again!*

Maybe I should buy lottery tickets.

Divine Secret: Sometimes Luck's Not a Lady. Sometimes She's an Evil Bee-Yotch.

Don't let my personal tale of chemo woe unnerve you. I may be Bad Luck Schleprock, the Flintstones character shadowed by a dark rain cloud, constantly stumbling into misfortune. But surely you are more of a Bam-Bam, smashing cancer with your caveman club. Talk to your health care provider about your personal risk factors. Chemotherapy can be scary, but for most people, the experience falls somewhere between tolerable and torturous, but not life-threatening.

Get Me Out of Here!

I'm jolted awake by a lightning bolt of terror. My heart thumps like a jackhammer.

Where are my kids? Are they okay?

All night long, I've been haunted by a nightmare that my children are missing. I can't find them, despite frantic searching.

It's dark outside, so I look at the clock. It's 6:30 a.m. I know I'm in the hospital, that the kids are home with Ryan, yet logic cannot quell the anxiety. My hands shake as if afflicted with Parkinson's. Panicking, even though it makes no sense, I reach for the phone.

Ryan picks up on the second ring.

"Is everyone okay? Are the kids okay?"

"Yes, honey. The kids are fine."

"You're sure?"

"Everything's under control. What's wrong, sweetie?"

"I had this…bad dream…thought I'd lost them."

"Don't worry, baby. It was just a nightmare. I'll be there soon."

I close my eyes, take deep, calming breaths, and let the relief sink in.

～

Surgeons continue to rotate in and out of my hospital room. The pain has subsided, but the antibiotics make me feel queasy. Ryan arrives after getting the kids off to school, so we call Mom.

"Hi, Mom. I'm, uh, in the hospital."

"The hospital?"

"Yeah, I had a bad reaction yesterday." I fill her in on the details.

"Why didn't you call me last night?"

"We didn't want you to worry."

"I'll pack and be there soon. But you should have called last night."

The rattle of food service carts in the hallway reminds me there'll be no pancakes and sausage delivered to my room. Not even a banana or yogurt. To alleviate the inflammation in my plumbing, I'm not allowed to eat anything.

The nurses tell me I'll soon be upgraded to the "ice-chip diet," meaning that for the next few days breakfast, lunch, and dinner will consist of—you guessed it—ice chips!

But, hey, it's bound to work better than the South Beach or Atkins diets.

> **Divine Secret: Have a back-up back-up plan.**
>
> It's one thing to plan for scheduled surgeries and treatments. But what if something happens without warning? Figure out who you can call and how you'll prioritize things in an emergency. Don't get so myopically focused on life's little details that you fail to see the bigger picture.

~

Bubbly Nurse Navigator stops in for a visit. But this time she's not wearing her pink hat or carrying pom-poms. "How are you feeling?"

"Not great, but better than I was."

"I heard no more chemo for you."

Her comment settles like a cold lump of oatmeal in my empty stomach.

"I thought so. It sounds strange, but I'm kind of disappointed I can't finish all the treatments."

"I know. But remember that your cancer was caught at an early stage. Chemo was more of a preventative measure."

"Yeah, but I really wanted one of those 'Farewell to Chemo' cakes."

"We can work something out."

After Bubbly Nurse Navigator leaves, I reflect on what's happened in the last few months. I think of the Mark Twain quote, "When ill luck begins, it does not come in sprinkles but in showers." *Yeah, it's been one hell of a downpour lately.*

~

As the days run together in an endless stretch, Ryan and Mom take turns coming to see me, bringing the kids by after school or in the evening. Neighbors and friends drop in, bearing fuzzy slippers and magazines. Pastors Barry and Lloyd visit, sharing prayers and encouragement. It seems that whenever I have a visitor, the scarf slips from my bald head, but I'm too weak to feel self-conscious.

I get to know the different nurses, who come in my room around the clock to check my vitals and change out the medication drips. My favorite is Angel Nurse, a tall, beautiful blonde who compliments me on my children.

"Your kids are really sweet," she says. "And so polite."

"Thank you." I laugh, glad she hasn't witnessed their loud burps or rude farts.

"They probably keep you busy."

"They do," I reply. "How about you? Any kids?"

"No." She looks away, then heads for the door. "Just press the call button if you need anything."

I'm surprised by her abrupt departure, but chalk it up to the demands of other patients.

In contrast, my least favorite person is Nurse Clueless, who tromps into my room at 3 a.m., turning on all the overhead

lights and talking loudly. She's a recent nursing school graduate, but why can't she enter quietly and carry a flashlight, like
the more experienced nurses?

After my troubling nightmare, I swear off Ambien. You
might think a hospital would be a good place to get some rest,
but you'd be wrong. At this point, it's not the pain that's keeping me up, it's the stupid IV machine. The damned thing won't
stop beeping! I drift off to sleep, but if I change my position in
the slightest, the IV unit emits a loud, piercing alarm. I never
get more than a short nap.

Periodically, a nurse injects a shot into my abdomen of a drug
that's supposed to raise my white cell count. The low-grade fever
continues. My bone marrow aches. My stomach spins. I've been
keeping a mental tally since my crash-landing in Cancerland,
and after receiving 50+ needle sticks for blood draws and injections, I'm now an official human pin cushion.

But the one bright spot is that whenever Angel Nurse is on
duty, she's willing to strike up a conversation.

"Your daughter? She's so cute! I'm guessing she's adopted,
right?"

"Yes. From China."

"How old was she when you got her?"

"Ten months. All four of us travelled to get her. It was an
amazing trip."

"That's good to hear. Not all adoptions go smoothly."

"True, but there are no guarantees, no matter how you add a
child to your family."

"Hmm," she says. "You're right."

"I can tell you, though, that I've met a lot of people with beautiful Chinese daughters."

~

As the days pass, I'm allowed to imbibe clear liquids, slowly
progressing to such haute cuisine as applesauce and the ubiq-
uitous green jello.

On one particularly bad night, my IV line kinks every few minutes, constantly setting off the shrill alarm. This machine is making me psychotic—I'm ready to destroy it with an axe, à la Jack Nicholson in *The Shining*. To make matters worse, Nurse Clueless has a cold and coughs on me every single time she comes in to adjust my IV monitor.

Perhaps a contagious employee should not work in the oncology ward? *Ya think?*

By the end of the week, I'm frustrated, restless, and so ready to go home. Bored, I shuffle back and forth down the hall, but I'm not allowed past the double doors. Trying to pass the time, I sit in the small, vacant visitor lounge, reading wrinkled magazines and drinking stale coffee.

Except for the shrill, repetitive noises of the medical equipment, the oncology ward stays very quiet. Though I never get more than a fleeting glimpse of other patients, I'm aware of their presence. Sometimes I hear the wheezy breathing of a silver-haired lady across the hall. Based on the number of big, tough cops visiting and wiping tears from their faces, there must be a fellow officer here. It's unnerving to realize some patients won't go home—at least not to their earthly abode.

It saddens me to think of dying here, beneath institutional hospital linens, surrounded by laminate cabinets and Styrofoam water pitchers, encircled by a blur of unfamiliar faces performing clinical tasks, tethered to this world by a tangle of cords.

My eyes water. I want to go home. *Now!*

But before Dr. Point Guard will release me, I have to prove I can swallow enormous antibiotic pills so the nurses can remove my IV. Huge, bitter, and chalky, they gag me every time I try to wash them down.

I'm as trapped as a prisoner in the jailhouse sick ward. *Somebody bake me a cake with a nail file inside, puhleze! I'll dig my way out!*

In the middle of the night when I can't sleep, big tears roll down my cheeks.

Only now am I starting to comprehend the fragility of health. Maybe my nightmare was a subconscious manifestation of my will to be here for my children. I reach into the drawer of my bedside table and pull out a *Gideon's Bible*.

I've never met a Gideon, but at this moment I'm intensely thankful for them. Their book is abridged, composed of the *New Testament*, along with *Psalms* and *Proverbs*. This shortened version makes sense; if, when in search of spiritual comfort, you started with *Genesis*, you might croak before getting past all the "begetting."

From weeks of Vacation Bible School during my childhood, I remember the 23rd Psalm:

Yea, though I walk through the valley of the shadow of death, I will fear no evil; For thou art with me. Thy rod and thy staff, they comfort me...

Angel Nurse walks into my room and sees that I'm crying. "What's wrong?"

"I-I-I can't go home until I can swallow my meds." I choke back a sob, holding up a gigantic pill.

"I'm sorry you're having a hard time." She straightens my blanket. "I don't usually tell my patients this, but I'm a survivor, too."

"You had breast cancer?"

"No, ovarian. Diagnosed in my 20s. Because of treatment, I can't bear children. It's hard, because I always wanted them."

She's so young! I would never have guessed. Now I understand why she's been so curious about adoption.

"After facing the disease myself, I decided I wanted to be an oncology nurse. Listen, I know this is hard. The stress can be overwhelming. But you're going to be okay."

I hang on her every word.

She writes something on a slip of paper and hands it to me. "I found these relaxation tapes—they really helped me cope."

"Thanks," I sniffle.

"You'll get through this. You will."

Angel Nurse pats my shoulder. Suddenly, I have a brainstorm, realizing exactly how to get those gigantic, yucky horse pills down. "Can you get me one of those margarine pods from the meal trays?"

"Sure. I'll be right back."

Borrowing Ryan's technique for slipping our dogs heartworm pills, I coat

Divine Secret: Sometimes the briefest interactions can be incredibly profound.

The "This is What Healing Looks Like" photograph transformed my attitude about hair loss. And by sharing her own experiences, Angel Nurse saved me from despair. Maybe I gave her hope that although she couldn't physically bear children, she could still be a mom. You never know how you might affect another's life with your words or deeds or how they might touch you.

the tablets until they're greased and slippery. I place them in my mouth and take a hurried gulp of ginger ale. *Success!*

Resource: Relaxation audios

Check out Belleruth Naparstek's array of audios you can download to relieve anxiety, inspire relaxation, and cope with treatments at healthjourneys.com.

Resource: Fertile Hope

This nonprofit, at fertilehope.org, provides reproductive information, support, and hope to people concerned about the risk of infertility after cancer treatment.

Buy One Surgery, Get One Free

October 2007

I'm thrilled when Dr. Point Guard signs my release papers a few days later. Ryan carries my overnight bag while an orderly pushes me in the hospital-mandated wheelchair. I feel like I've been sprung from Alcatraz.

Minutes after arriving home, my friend Kathleen drops Larissa off after her Girl Scout pajama party.

"Mommy! You're home!" She runs to the couch to embrace me.

"I've got my pajamas on, too," I say. "We can have our own little PJ party."

We snuggle on the couch, watching a cartoon, while I inhale the sweetness of the moment.

After she falls asleep, I log onto *CaringBridge* and update my blog, bragging about my amazing weight loss results from the "Ice-Chip Diet."

∼

After several weeks of recovery, I find my dance card filled as I waltz to various medical appointments. Jolly General Surgeon, a tall man with a deep guffaw, recommends surgery to repair my damaged intestines—once my immune system is strong enough—and tells me I'll be in the hospital for a week.

Not again! Seriously, the hospital should issue frequent customer cards like the airlines do. Surely I'd collect enough points to redeem a Hammacher Schlemmer gadget.

Over the next few days, I think about adding a second surgical procedure. I've read recent oncology studies investigating how medically-induced menopause—either permanently by surgery or temporarily by medications or injections—might help ward off recurrence in women who are strongly estrogen-positive.

Divine Secret: Deep inside, we are more alike than different.

Rather than night-vision goggles, cancer has given me soul-vision spectacles. We may appear separated from others by nationality, race, age, religion, education, or income bracket, but cancer, or any serious illness, is a profound equalizer. All of us—Wall Street wizards, African goat-herders, European countesses, school lunch ladies—share the same raw, human experiences: fear, grief, love, hope.

Should I get my ovaries yanked? While I'm already under the knife?

Not all Pink Sisters want this. Many younger women still long for children and would rule out this option. And not all oncologists agree on the risks versus benefits. I don't know if I would pursue an oophorectomy if I didn't need surgery anyway.

Yet for my situation, it's not that drastic. At age 45, I'm done having children, not far from the age of natural menopause, and extremely (95%) estrogen-positive. I won't miss those erratic visits from Aunt Flo, who always gives me a menstrual migraine as a hostess gift.

When I bring up the subject with Dr. Point Guard, he agrees it's something worth considering.

I am a bargain shopper extraordinaire. Two surgeries for the price of one!

～

Divine Secret: Medical guidelines are constantly changing.

Oncologists keep up with the constant stream of new studies and scientific discoveries, making changes in treatment recommendations when appropriate. Ask your doctor about the latest news from some of the clinical trials, like the ones studying ovarian suppression and adjuvant therapies.

Now I have to find a gynecologist to perform this surgery, since Jolly General Surgeon does not operate on girly bits. And Calming Gynecologist doesn't have operating privileges at the hospital where Jolly General Surgeon practices.

What a logistical nightmare. Why can't the medical community follow the same rules as the old *Operation* board game, where any player can pluck out any part?

A neighbor recommends Vivacious Gynecologist, a middle-aged blonde with a warm, friendly bedside manner. At her office, we spend ten minutes discussing my health history. I can't help but think she can empathize with the challenges of fertility, childbirth, and menopause easier than a male physician.

I fill her in on my breast cancer diagnosis. We discuss reconstruction surgery, and I tell her I'm considering having a prophylactic mastectomy on the left side.

"Not everyone would agree with me," she confides. "But if I was diagnosed with breast cancer, I'd want a bilateral, too."

She brings up the pros and cons of removing various girly parts. "With your sub-type of cancer, estrogen is not your friend. Taking out the ovaries and fallopian tubes would shut down the major producer of this hormone in your body. And since tamoxifen increases your risk of uterine cancer, you should consider having your uterus removed as well. I'd recommend a hysterectomy with bilateral salpingo-oophorectomy."

Wow, a medical term longer than supercalifragilisticexpialidocious!

"On the other hand," she continues, "estrogen provides certain benefits. You need to pay special attention to your heart and bone health."

"Diet, calcium supplements, and weight-bearing exercise, right?"

"Yes. I have to warn you, though," she says, pursing her lips and peering over the top of her glasses. "Removing your ovaries will slam-dunk you into menopause. And it won't be safe to take any type of hormone replacement."

I nod, resigned. With my sky-high ER/PR+ status, hormone replacement will be contraindicated *whenever* I go through menopause—whether naturally or surgically-induced.

But how bad will the symptoms be? Some women describe the transition as a minor bump while others find it a major upheaval. After all, the shared female experience of hot flashes, night sweats, and mood swings inspired the catchy lyrics for *Menopause the Musical: The Hilarious Celebration of Women and the Change.* So there's got to be something to it.

Leaving her office, I think about the tradeoffs: whenever you deal with one health issue, the side effects of treatment cause other problems to pop up like a game of *Whack-a-Mole.*

Divine Secret: There are trade-offs with every procedure or treatment.

I know firsthand that chemotherapy's toxicity is a two-edged sword. It may get rid of the cancer but can cause neuropathy or other unwelcome residual effects. But the same concept applies when considering surgery. There may be benefits, but there can also be serious drawbacks.

~

It takes time to fully grasp the circumstances of my emergency hospitalization. Caught up in the desire to retain normalcy, Ryan and I misjudged the situation. Dr. Point Guard seemed so calm and reassuring, that once the pain was addressed, I didn't understand enough to worry. But looking back at that night, I'm stunned we didn't call Mom immediately or ask a neighbor to watch the kids.

Curious, I google statistics on patients who experience a similar complication while undergoing chemo. I feel a chill as I read of possible dire outcomes. For a few scary hours, I was in jeopardy. Like a soldier injured not on the battlefield, but in a traffic accident while home on leave, I was focusing on the obvious enemy—cancer—and was ambushed by my most recent health crisis.

Divine Secret: Don't wring your hands in regret, second-guessing medical decisions.

You make your treatment choices, but you can't control the outcome. You take your best shot, based on the information you have at the time. Sometimes your decision is a slam-dunk or a buzzer-beater that clinches victory. But sometimes it's an air ball, a complete miss.

In hindsight, some would say chemo was not the best choice for me. Maybe, if my treatment path had been more straightforward—a lumpectomy with clean margins, followed up by radiation—I would have been comfortable forgoing chemo. But after discovering more than one tumor, needing a mastectomy, then facing a Stage IV scare, I don't think there is any way I would have made a different decision.

~

Since I parted ways with Doctor Doofus, I have to find a new primary care provider, per my insurance policy. Dr. Earnest is a tall, slender man with a pleasant demeanor. After shaking my hand, he squints at his computer screen.

"I've spent a lot of time reading your history. The hospital has been setting up a network where all doctors treating the same patient have access to shared information."

He speaks in a very slow, calm manner, sort of like a hostage negotiator. I'm a little paranoid: *Did Doctor Doofus flag my medical records with a warning? Beware unbalanced, volatile patient.* Not sure I like the idea of doctors adding their subjective comments to my file. It's a little intimidating, like the warning you get as a kid: that transgressions will go on your "permanent record."

After an exam and discussion, Dr. Earnest writes me a prescription for a drug used to treat hot flashes in women who can't take hormone replacement therapy. He explains that although it's an anti-depressant, Effexor helps minimize the hot flashes.

"Get it filled right away. Start taking it now to build up in your system. Some of my patients have had a miserable time with menopause."

Is it really that bad? Well, if nothing else, at least I'll be in a good mood whenever I need to stick my head in the freezer.

So far, I'm impressed with Dr. Earnest's bedside manner. But as he leaves the room, he gives me a warning. "Breast cancer is tricky." He shakes his head in dismay. "With many cancers, you can feel confident you've beaten it at the five-year mark, but with breast cancer, it can recur ten, fifteen, twenty years after diagnosis."

Thanks, doc! Just what I wanted to hear.

~

Following our Halloween tradition, the moms in our cul-de-sac sit outside in folding chairs, chatting while we hand out candy. During the first hour, we stay busy with a procession of miniature witches, ninjas, and fairies.

My neighbor Sarah offers me a glass of wine.

"Thanks!" I say, reaching for the plastic cup. "I'm off the pain meds so I can enjoy a little vino."

"How are you doing?"

"I've got several weeks of freedom. Then back to the hospital for more surgery."

"I'm sorry."

"Thanks. But this surgery will be different. The tumors are already gone."

"Thank God."

"It's going to be a long process." I unwrap a mini-Snickers. "Reconstruction means several more operations."

"Wow."

A tiny Cinderella approaches with a pink pumpkin. Her mom greets me. "Hi, Joanna. How are you doing?"

Still fixated on all the "Save the Date" blocks in my mental calendar, I blurt out the first thing that comes to my chemo-addled, chardonnay-buzzed mind. "Well, I'm going to enjoy the free time I have left."

Turning pale, the mom hurries away before I realize what I've done.

*Ack! I'm such an idiot; I meant the free time **before heading back to surgery!***

The next day, I send her an apologetic e-mail explaining my remark.

Divine Secret: You get a Stupid Pass, too.

We all make dumb comments. If you insert your foot in your mouth as often as I do, you'll need an entire notepad of Stupid Passes!

Copy and clip as needed:

Stupid Pass

Name:_____

Date:_____

Comment:_____

_____

Stupid Pass

Name:_____

Date:_____

Comment:_____

_____

Stupid Pass

Name:_____

Date:_____

Comment:_____

_____

Do I Get a Frequent Patient Card?

November 2007

We enjoy a pleasant Thanksgiving with Ryan's extended family, and then I prepare for my next round of surgery. Mom packs up her bags once again and settles into Alex's room. I can't thank her enough for all the time she has spent here helping us out.

At my pre-op anesthesiology appointment, the nurse asks about my experiences undergoing general anesthesia.

"I have a lot of nausea when I wake up. It was pretty bad after my mastectomy."

"We don't want that to happen again," she assures me. "We'll give you plenty of anti-nausea medications."

"Thank you!"

"Any allergies to rubber or latex?"

"No."

"Any medication allergies?"

"No, not that I know of."

"Any other allergies? To food products? Anything at all?"

"Well, cats," I say, waiting for her to crack a smile. "But I don't suppose that would be a problem in the O.R."

Serious Nurse continues going over her checklist, making sure she gives me the usual pre-surgical warnings. "Nothing to eat or drink after midnight."

"Okay."

"Remember to shower with Hibiclens soap."

"I will."

"Don't use any hairspray on the day of surgery."

"O...kay."

I struggle to keep a straight face. My medical record has "CANCER" scrawled all over it, probably in flashing lights. *And didn't she notice me tug the wig in place just minutes ago?* But with my au naturel peach fuzz hairdo, foregoing Aqua Net is *so* not a problem.

~

The night before surgery, I update my *CaringBridge* page, spreading a little white lie: "My doctors have decreed no visitors except immediate family." I enjoyed holding court during previous hospital stay-cations, but I want a little privacy while my digestive system reboots.

Waking up in the recovery room, I'm extremely sleepy. But at least I'm not sick to my stomach. Ryan tries to tell me the surgery went well, but his words seem fuzzy and hard to understand.

Throughout the first days of my hospital stay, I remain in a drug-induced haze, on more powerful medications than after my mastectomy. Between visits from Ryan, Mom, and the kids, I take frequent naps. Unable to remember anything, I keep re-reading the same magazine.

Peeking under my unflattering hospital gown—*Vera Wang, are you listening?*—I discover a vertical scar of several inches, as well as some smaller incisions. My body looks like a roadmap!

After several days of nothing but ice chips on the menu, I'm thrilled with my tray of beef bouillon and the reliable green jello. But couldn't food services throw caution to the wind and give me a bowl of red—even orange—wiggly gelatin? Yet, on the plus side, when it comes to accommodations, I've been upgraded to first class—in the new wing of the hospital, my room outfitted with a flat-screen TV. But just my luck—the one time I have a guilt-free pass to watch all the TV I could possibly want, the writers are on strike. There's nothing on but re-runs.

With encouragement from the nurses, I put on my slippers and, pushing the IV pole along, walk the halls. The floor is laid out in a rectangular formation, with a nurses station at each end. The mood is cheerier here than in the oncology ward—no surprise—yet I rarely see or hear any patients. Many of the rooms are fitted with larger doors and bigger beds, designed for bariatric patients undergoing gastric bypass surgery. I imagine most of them are happy to be here, ready to start living a healthier lifestyle.

The staff nurses and nursing assistants are nice and helpful. Because they've yet to imbibe the "Service Excellence" corporate kool-aid, there are no practiced spiels, no names scribbled on my whiteboard. Can't say I miss them. *But who knows, maybe they've been talking about "Service Excellence" all along, and I'm too doped up to remember?*

Anyway, doctors get plenty of kudos, but it's the nurses who administer most of the patient care. Like teachers, sometimes their contributions are overlooked or undervalued. However, there's one particular nurse who keeps pestering me. Potty Patrol Nurse is constantly checking on my bathroom habits, warning me I can't go home until I make doo-doo. I feel like a toddler trying to earn a Care Bear sticker.

Divine Secret: Healing takes time.

Everyone wants the fastest route out of Cancerland, but sometimes you have a detour. You may encounter unanticipated bumps in the road that require a delay of surgery or treatment. Try to be a patient patient.

To pass the time, I watch reality shows on TLC. Often overwhelmed with just three kids, I can't imagine trading places with Michelle Duggar, the devoutly religious mom with pioneer-style dresses and fourteen kids, all given names beginning with "J."

I tune into *Jon & Kate Plus 8*, a repeat episode where the kids go to a

Fourth of July parade. I hate to admit it, but I'm really more of a cranky Kate Gosselin than a blissful Michelle Duggar.

~

After a week, once I've demonstrated my bathroom prowess, the nurses buy me a Magical Mermaid Barbie and take me to Baskin-Robbins for a banana split. No, not really. But I do get to go home, an even better reward.

Once my incisions heal enough that I can wear jeans comfortably, it's obvious I've lost weight, though I'm still not exactly thin. Worried about my depleted energy level, my figure-conscious Mom—who once gave me her "extra" copy of the South Beach Diet book—encourages me to put more butter and cheese on my baked potato.

Divine Secret: Chewing gum can jump-start your digestive system.

Several medical studies have shown that chewing gum in the days following surgery gets your digestive juices flowing. Ask your doctor about this.

Recovery:

Slacker Survivor

Feeling Hot, Hot, Hot

December 2007

Vivacious Gynecologist (the physician who removed my girly parts) and Dr. Earnest, my new primary care provider, weren't joking about menopause. With my personal thermostat completely off kilter, neither Ryan nor I get much sleep. I kick the blankets off one minute, then pull them up the next. The hot flashes turn my complexion beet red. My internal space heater is cranked to full blast. I'm melting into a puddle, just like the Wicked Witch of the West.

Before long, I'm managing my post-surgical pain with Tylenol during the day and prescription meds at night to sleep. Yet due to my new hormonal status, I wake up every morning with sodden hair and tangled sheets.

Mom has been such a trooper, taking care of the family, doing the laundry, driving me to appointments, providing moral support. But I know she's tired of living out of a suitcase and needs a break.

So we ask Ryan's oldest sister, Dianne, to come for a week. Not only is she wonderful at looking after the kids and keeping the house running, she's a pleasant companion, sharing wisdom from her adventures in parenting. As the days progress, I feel stronger, so she drives me to the mall for Christmas shopping. I walk gingerly, allowing her to carry the packages, but it feels great to be out of the house. My slow-motion stroll around the mall feels like a victory lap.

Summer has slipped into fall without my noticing the change of seasons, so I'm jarred by all the holiday decorations. Excited children line up to get photos with Santa. Every store is decked with greenery, blinking lights, glittery bows. The aisles are crowded with seasonal retailers such as the reliable Hickory Farms display of sausage and cheese baskets, as well as local artists hawking hand-painted ornaments.

On a mission to find something fun to wear to a neighbor's party, I browse through racks of cheesy holiday sweaters. As I feel a surge of warmth, followed by dampness at the back of my neck, I realize I'd burn up in a bulky cardigan or high-necked pull-over. Dianne and I visit several shops until I find a short-sleeved silky red blouse, festive yet cool.

⁓

By the time Dianne returns home, I've regained some energy. I'm happy to be back to doing laundry and cooking, although Ryan and the boys are missing the four- and five-star meals.

The last few months have been tough, but I'm starting to feel the Christmas spirit. Like we do every year, Ryan and I sit down and agree on a gift-buying budget. But this time, we completely ignore it. Jubilant to put cancer behind us, we go on a shopping spree, buying the kids everything on their lists, plus the latest videogame console for the boys and a gigantic stuffed horse for Larissa. Surrounded by holiday cheer, I take the kids to buy toys for a local charity and canned goods for a food pantry.

⁓

The anti-depressant Dr. Earnest prescribed for my hot flashes doesn't seem to be working yet, so whenever I'm in the car, I crank up the AC and learn forward, putting my face close to the vents. It might be snowing outside, but it's tropical summer in

Joanna-ville. Complaints begin immediately.

"Mommy, I'm cold," Larissa whines.

"Put on your sweater, sweetie."

"Dang, Mom," complains Alex, "this feels like an igloo on wheels!"

"You're a boy scout. You'll survive."

"Wow, your face is red, Mom!" crows Nick. "You look like a tomato!"

As payback, I lower the temperature several more degrees and start belting out lyrics to the Pussycat Dolls' song: *"Don't cha wish your girlfriend was hot like me, don't cha wish..."*

All three kids groan in embarrassment, once again mortified by their crazy mother.

∿

Over the school break, Mom and I take Alex and Nick to see *I Am Legend*, the new Will Smith action movie. The plot hurls an ugly curveball.

The villains Will Smith battles?

Zombified cancer patients!

I sit in the cinema and watch weak, ravaged cancer survivors with patchy hair and ghostly complexions transform into blood-thirsty, homicidal zombies.

Enough with the cancer, already.

Afterwards, we squeeze some laughs out of the plot twist. I spend the next few days sneaking up on the boys, surprising them with my eerie "cancer zombie" voice and fearsome expression.

∿

We spend Christmas with my folks in the mountains. Especially grateful this year, we participate in a candlelight church service, unwrap gifts stacked under the tree, and feast on a roasted turkey with all the trimmings. I've selected a special gift for Ryan,

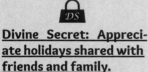

**Divine Secret: Appreci-
ate holidays shared with
friends and family.**

It's not about the gifts,
the decorations, or the
meal. The most precious
gift that you can give and
receive is love.

a silver photo frame engraved with words from a Robert Browning poem—"grow old along with me, the best is yet to be"—and he fusses at me for making him teary in front of everyone. All of us are teary, our emotions ragged from the drama since my diagnosis. It turns out to be a wonderful holiday, just not a perfect Currier & Ives one, especially when Nick cranks up the volume on Larissa's pink Barbie electric guitar and refuses to stop playing it, turning us all into Grinches.

I'm a Middle-Aged Groupie

January 2008

I can barely contain my excitement. Beth, my BFF from Texas, is flying out for a visit.

"Guess what, guys?" I say, dishing out plates of spaghetti. "Beth's taking me to the Matchbook Twenty concert. Bought us second-row seats!"

Alex rolls his eyes. "It's Matchbox, not Matchbook."

"I knew that," I lie. "Ooh, maybe the band will pull me on stage to dance," I tease. "Like Bruce Springsteen did with Courtney Cox in the 'Born in the U.S.A.' video!"

"Stop, Mom!" Nick says. "Promise us you won't do anything like that."

"Yes," pleads Alex. "Try to act normal."

~

A few days later, I pick up Beth at the airport. She's wearing a red coat, her locks now shoulder length and chestnut brown, rather than long and highlighted.

"Your hair looks great," I tell her.

"So does yours!" she replies, admiring my glossy blonde wig.

"Thanks. It's better than the stubble underneath."

"You could totally pull off the bald Star Trek lady look."

On the drive home, we catch up, talking about our families and a trip we're planning. The last few months have been tough for Beth, too, with her dad and brother battling serious illnesses. We sit up late, sharing stories and laughing.

~

The following evening, we dress for the concert. I'm wearing dark jeans with a silky black blouse. I bought the top during a frustrating shopping trip, hunting for something cute that would conceal the clone without looking dowdy. Beth's wearing a black lace shirt and denim skirt.

"Love your boots," I say.

"Gotta look good for my boyfriend on stage."

"Who cares that he's married to a gorgeous model?"

"He'll see me in the audience. Realize I'm his true soulmate."

"You're starting to sound stalker-ish."

"No, way!"

"Yes, way. But I'm excited, too. Can't wait to hear Dave Thomas."

"Jo, it's *Rob* Thomas," she sighs. "Dave is the Wendy's guy."

"Chemo-brain!" I say, trying to cover my gaffe. "Tonight's going to be fun."

"And we're in need of some major fun."

"Maybe there'll be some cute guys at the VIP party," I hint. Beth is attractive, funny, and outgoing, but hasn't dated much since her divorce.

"When and if I go out, it'll be with someone younger." She shakes her head. "Guys our age are no fun. Too boring and set in their ways."

"Like *my* husband?" I give her a sly grin.

"No, Ryan's a keeper. Even if he keeps close tabs on the pennies."

"Remember that time we all went to the beach? And he insisted there was no reason to stay in an oceanfront hotel when we could get two, *perfectly good, free* reward rooms?"

"Who cares if we had to drive twenty minutes to the beach rather than walk barefoot from the lobby? At least we got yummy cinnamon rolls at the breakfast buffet."

"And a lovely sunset view of the asphalt parking lot." We laugh.

"Hey, we can't dis Ryan. How many guys would take time off so their wife could vacation with a friend?"

True, that!

~

We're standing outside the arena, shivering. Food service vendors and souvenir hawkers are setting up tables, but no one will let us in the lobby. I wave to a security guard, but he shakes his head. Despite the laminated card around my neck, I'm not feeling very VIP-ish.

To pass the time, I check out the people waiting with us. One guy has ear studs the size of poker chips, freakishly elongating his earlobes. His date has normal-looking ears, but several nose piercings. One strikingly pretty woman, with raven-black hair accentuated by a bold white streak, flirts with her date. A tall, rangy woman in skintight jeans and cowboy boots stands beside us, smoking a cigarette. She has a flinty expression and unfortunate complexion.

"Have you seen Matchbox Twenty before?" Beth asks.

"Hell, yeah!" answers Cowgirl Groupie. "Three times in the last two months." She takes a long drag from her cigarette. "And I'm always up real close. Don't care how much the tickets cost. I live for this."

Finally, a party hostess escorts us to the VIP reception. She gives each of us two coupons for alcoholic beverages. Famished, I head for the appetizer spread. Since I'm the driver, I decide to have only one glass of wine and give my extra drink ticket to Beth.

"Ooh, I really want to win something!" Beth says, as we look over the collection of stadium blankets and t-shirts designated as door prizes.

"I could share my story with the party hostess. Ditch my wig and put on a bandanna."

"Yeah, play that cancer card!"

"No, not worth it for a measly t-shirt."

~

An hour later, we're escorted to our seats in the middle of the second row. Security guards stand watch in case the crowd gets rowdy. Pretty Skunk-Haired Girl sits directly in front of us, while her companion is in the third row, next to Earlobe Guy and Pierced Nose Girl.

"What's the deal?" asks Beth. "Why aren't you sitting together?"

"I wanted to be as close to the stage as possible," she replies, flipping her hair. "But I could only get one front-row ticket, so he's in row three." We learn he's a graphic artist and that they travel to comic book conventions, where she dresses up in a sexy superhero costume while he signs autographs for geeky fans.

"How old are you?" Beth asks Comic Book Dude.

"Thirty-four."

"How about you?" She points to Earlobe Guy.

"Twenty-seven."

She nudges me. "See, I told you!"

A couple takes the empty seats beside Beth. While the stage-hands set up, we learn the wife's a realtor and the husband's a homebuilder. He tells us they used to work together, and he'd make up excuses to call her before working up the nerve to ask for a date.

Blonde Realtor glances at Beth's lanyard. "Is that a backstage pass?"

"No, VIP package. We got a wine and cheese reception, t-shirts, poster, USB of tonight's concert, plus customized iPods. But unfortunately no backstage access."

"Sorry," says Hunky Homebuilder. "I didn't pay for VIP extras."

"She splurged," I say, trying to make the guy feel better.

"She had cancer," Beth blurts.

"I'm so sorry!" Blonde Realtor replies.

"Thanks, but I'm fine now."

"Doesn't she look great?" Beth chirps. "Can you believe she's wearing a wig? That she's bald underneath?"

Okay, I'm starting to cringe. Beth should slow down on the vino. Good thing I'm the designated driver tonight.

Opening act Alanis Morissette takes the stage. Everyone is on their feet. The concert experience is totally different up close where you can see every expression, every gesture. After a few high-intensity songs, Alanis turns the mood mellow, perching on a stool and strapping on her acoustic guitar. Following her lead, the audience sits down. Beth went to the concession stand, and I realize she hasn't returned.

"Did your friend leave you?" Blonde Realtor asks, a worried look on her face.

"No, she'll be back."

She pats Beth's empty seat. "Come sit beside us."

This woman feels sorry for me.

"She'll be back soon," I reassure her. Beth shows up a few minutes later.

"Sorry, I got caught up in the moment." She hands me a soda. "Spent a little time dancing in the aisles."

"No problem," I say. "Although our new friends thought you ditched me."

"I'd never do that!" she insists, turning to Blonde Realtor. "Joanna's my BFF."

The lights come on as stagehands set up for Matchbox Twenty. Beth is getting goofier by the moment.

"How old are you?" she asks Hunky Homebuilder.

"Thirty-eight."

"See!" shouts Beth. "I told you! Any guy I find attractive is younger!"

Hunky Homebuilder blushes. Blonde Realtor giggles. I laugh so hard I start to cough.

Skunk-Haired Girl turns around to chat. Her boyfriend's gone to the concession stand, so she shares her relationship issues. "I can't get him to commit."

Wow, some experiences are universal. Even women with dragon tattoos and metal-studded leather chokers have to deal with their guys' commitment issues.

"We've been living together for two years," she explains. "But he wants to keep his options open. He still dates other women. I hate when he brings them home."

"That's terrible!"

"What a jerk," Beth says. "You don't need him."

"That's right," I add. "You're a lovely girl! You need to find someone who'll treat you with respect."

Now I'm giving Skunk-Haired Girl dating advice?

Comic Book Dude returns, asking us to pass a drink to his girlfriend. Beth and I roll our eyes.

"You can cross him off the list," I mumble.

"Definitely."

Rob Thomas takes the stage and Matchbox Twenty launches into their newest hit song. The crowd goes crazy. We're standing, cheering, moving in time to the music. Rob Thomas stares into the first few rows. It seems as if he's looking right at me, his gorgeous blue eyes peering into my soul. The feeling is intoxicating and electrifying. I can see the stubble on his chin, the diamond stud in his ear, the beads of sweat forming on his forehead.

I understand the groupie mentality!

The band starts the electric guitar riffs for their hit song "Bent." Then the red-haired musician in the preppy blazer and high-top sneakers stops playing. His frustration mounting, he attempts to adjust his guitar strings. Somebody should tell him Angus Young from AC/DC wants his schoolboy uniform back. The audience is silent, tension building. The guitarist hurls his instrument offstage, cursing out a stage-hand.

After a few awkward seconds, the chastened roadie hands over a back-up guitar. As the music re-starts, everyone stands up and dances. *I'm elated. I'm alive, done with cancer treatment! Hanging out with my BFF!* My body's scarred, but my spirit is soaring. I float up with the music, my blood throbbing in time with the beat. Rob looks at me again, his eyes laser-like and piercing. Caught up in the moment, I blow him a kiss, like a nutcase stalker. He recoils and looks away.

I'm having a blast, but I'm not really a groupie. I'd never throw my lingerie on stage. After all, my tummy control granny pants aren't exactly sexy. And if I threw my post-mastectomy bra and clone, poor Rob Thomas could end up with a concussion.

Divine Secret: Let the good times roll!

Break out of your comfort zone and have some much-needed fun! Spend time hanging out with friends and family. Love and laughter are a salve for your soul.

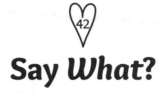

Say *What?*

As the weeks pass, the gloomy winter weather makes it hard to stay upbeat. For now, I'm done with surgery. Reconstruction can wait; our family needs a break. I wish my body could have tolerated all my chemo sessions. I didn't exactly kick cancer's butt, but maybe I whacked it upside the head with my handbag.

The Matchbox Twenty concert with Beth was an emotional high, but now I'm swimming against a riptide of depression. I miss finding cards and packages in the mailbox, starting to empathize with those troubled souls with Munchausen's syndrome, who make up ailments for attention. I can't find my way back to normal. My mood gets darker each day, as I continue to get knocked down in tidal waves of bad news.

First, a college friend dies following a massive stroke. A former high school valedictorian, Sandra was brainy enough to be a rocket scientist, but her love for children inspired her to become a teacher and librarian. At age 43, with a devoted husband and two young children, she had a strong faith and one of the kindest hearts I've ever known. With curly blonde hair and crystal blue eyes, Central Casting couldn't have found a better angel. I buy sympathy cards for her family, filling the blank spaces with my memories of Sandra.

*The world was a better place with her **here**. Why did this happen?*

~

Weighed down with bleak emotions, I don't have the energy to pick up the phone. As I spend hours watching mindless TV, certain shows meld with my reality. I start thinking of the ladies of *The View* as personal pals, creating my own Fantasy Friendship League. In my mind, I share snarky jokes and martinis with Joy Behar, browse through Rosie O'Donnell's adoption scrapbooks, go shoe shopping with Elisabeth Hasselbeck, and listen in awe as Barbara Walters recounts fascinating career anecdotes.

But in real life, I can't summon the energy to invite a friend for coffee or schedule a lunch date. I'm not motivated to read, though books have always been a passion. It's a gargantuan effort to go to the grocery store. I hide out in pajamas all day and don't get dressed or put on lipstick until minutes before the afternoon school bus arrives. Aside from taking daily medication, I'm done with cancer treatment. *Shouldn't I be happy?*

Divine Secret: It takes time to find your "new normal."

One thing cancer survivors are rarely warned about is that the time following treatment can be the toughest of all emotionally. It's easier to be positive while you have an engaged support system of friends and family as well as frequent attention from medical personnel. But once treatment stops, everyone expects you to return to your former self. That may not happen.

~

One cold, dreary day, Mom calls. "I've got something to tell you." Her voice sounds strained. "You'd better sit down."

"What's going on?" I feel an icy spike of apprehension.

"You're not going to believe this. I've been diagnosed with breast cancer, too."

What?
What did she just say? Not cancer, not Mom!

"No! This can't be happening." I feel dizzy. We've become so close. I couldn't bear to lose her.

"I can't believe it, either! But I'm going to be okay."

This is stunning news. There's *no* history of cancer in our family. And now, both of us diagnosed months apart?

I feel winded, as if I've taken an uppercut to my ribs. "How did you find out? What have they said?"

"I had a clean mammogram just a few months ago. But one morning I noticed an inverted nipple, so I called my gynecologis. She ordered a diagnostic mammogram, which showed calcifications. They looked like tiny white stars."

"Are you having a biopsy?"

"Done. Confirmed DCIS, Ductal Carcinoma In Situ."

"Why didn't you tell me?"

"Look who's talking! You didn't tell me anything until after *your* biopsy. But I've thought it over and decided to get a lumpectomy. The doctor says I'll need radiation but not chemo."

Though crushed to hear her diagnosis, I'm relieved it's DCIS, also known as Stage 0. Breast cancer stinks no matter what stage, but if you're going to get it, Stage 0 is the best, since the malignant cells, still contained within the ducts, are not yet invasive or capable of spreading elsewhere. I'm grateful she has an excellent prognosis, but hate that she's dealing with this.

Yet one thing I've learned from my Pink Sisters is that DCIS can be very tricky and diffuse, meaning the patient may need multiple excisions or even a mastectomy to remove all affected tissue.

"Ask the surgeon for a breast MRI," I suggest. "It can show the extent of abnormal areas of DCIS better than a mammogram or ultrasound. I'm going to e-mail you an article I just read. Print it out and take it to your next appointment."

"Thank you, Doctor Joanna."

I make myself sound strong and encouraging, but after we hang up, I cry. I suspect she probably does, too.

~

Mom calls back a few days later, frustrated. "I'm not happy with the surgeon who did my biopsy. Or his office staff."

"What's going on?"

"Well, you know it was the physician assistant who told me the biopsy results were positive for DCIS. But the doctor hasn't called. His receptionist told me he's on vacation and won't be back for another week."

"So his office confirmed you had DCIS, but is now leaving you hanging?"

"Yes. And the receptionist was pretty snippy. She said I'd have to wait until my appointment to speak with him. And that the earliest opening they had was in two weeks."

"You're kidding. Is he an oncology surgeon?"

"No, a general surgeon. I told her I was wondering if I needed to see an oncologist. And she said the doctor would decide and then they would schedule an appointment if I needed one."

"Wow."

Apparently, Rude Receptionist needs an entire pitcher of the "Service Excellence" kool-aid.

~

Hard to believe Mom's facing cancer so soon after my diagnosis. I try to keep busy but some days all I want to do is sleep.

She calls back several days later. "Well, I finally spoke with the surgeon."

"What did he say about the breast MRI?"

Divine Secret: Sometimes life keeps throwing rotten tomatoes.

Okay, you've dealt with cancer. But now your spouse loses his job? Your kid is having trouble in school? Your parents are having health problems? Alas, life is not fair.

"That he wouldn't order it because it's too expensive."

"Really? Would he say that if it were *his* wife or daughter?"

"I've decided to find a different doctor. It's my body! I should have a say in the decision-making process. I talked to my gynecologist and she's given me a referral to a surgeon who specializes in women's cancer."

"Good for you! I agree."

As they say, the apple doesn't fall far from the tree.

A Brand New Healthy Me

January 2008

One chilly morning, Hannah, Liz, and I linger over coffee.

"Would you be interested in signing up for the Komen Race?" Liz asks. "There's one coming up in May. I'll do it with you."

Her question catches me off guard. I can't imagine running unless I'm being chased by a rabid dog or hungry bear.

"I don't know. Maybe." I've lost weight—albeit not in a healthy, points-counting Weight Watchers style—but I don't have much stamina or energy. While I've been stuck in Cancerland, Liz, however, has become an avid runner. She looks fabulous, like a contemporary Snow White, slender with a porcelain complexion and glossy black hair.

"I'll do it, too," chimes in Hannah, adding that our friend Winona from playgroup would probably want to join us.

"Not everyone runs," adds Liz. "You could walk or jog."

Hmm, in my condition, running's highly unlikely, jogging's questionable. But I could walk.

"Really? You'd do it with me? That might be fun."

∼

Using the upcoming race as motivation to adopt a healthier lifestyle, I brainstorm ideas. Shop more carefully. Avoid foods with suspected carcinogens. Grow pesticide-free vegetables. Buy eggs from hormone-free chickens. Raise goats in my backyard.

Scratch that last idea; our neighborhood association would have a hissy fit.

However, I won't go full-tilt "earth mother." No dreadlocks or strictly vegan diet for me. I'm a terrible cook. Too many of my culinary experiments have involved smoke alarms. But I can stop microwaving frozen, prepackaged lasagnas and buying meals from fast-food pick-up windows.

Fired with enthusiasm, I visit a specialty grocery store to purchase organic, healthy items. As I fill my cart, I try not to be discouraged by the anorexic chickens and bruised apples.

Back home, I unload my shopping bags, stocking the pantry with an array of snacks. Nick opens a box of whole wheat oatmeal raisin cookies.

"Blech! These taste like cardboard."

"Keep an open mind. You might develop a liking for them."

"Why'd you buy all this strange stuff?"

"We need to start eating healthier."

"Then maybe you could buy the *unfrosted* Pop-Tarts."

~

I decide to start actually working out at the YMCA, not just paying the monthly membership fee. At my first visit, I wander around confused, like a lost little kid. There's a step class going on, but the choreography seems far too challenging. Innately clumsy, I was always the last kid picked for kickball. The water aerobics class looks like fun, but it might not build my stamina quickly enough for the race. Plus, I'm not keen on wearing a bathing suit.

Intimidated by the hulking fitness machines, I walk over to the free weight area. I'm wary of lymphedema, the swelling of your arm and hand that can happen after lymph node removal.

Some experts warn survivors not to bear too much weight or do push-ups with the affected arm. Others believe that moderate weight-lifting is perfectly fine. *I hate conflicting opinions! For just once, can't all the experts agree?*

I decide to start on a bike and grab a magazine. Twenty minutes later, I find myself engrossed in an article, still pedaling at the lowest speed, not working up one bead of sweat. I put the magazine away and hop on a treadmill. Tightening my bandanna so it won't slip off, I walk briskly, even jog a few minutes before I feel winded.

I go again the next day.

And the next.

A gold star for me!

~

About a week later, Mom undergoes a lumpectomy. As she recovers, we keep our fingers crossed that her pathology report will show clear margins, meaning she won't need a re-excision.

Mom switched surgeons and really likes the new guy. Says his office is warm and homey, with rocking chairs and hot tea, rather than cold and clinical. And the nurses and office staff are helpful and nice. Most importantly, he spent over an hour talking to her and Pop at the first appointment, making sure all their questions were answered.

~

After another morning spent at the Y, I drive by the pharmacy to pick up a prescription refill. I think I'm starting to crush on Cute Pharmacy Dude, even though I'm old enough to be his— uh—older sister.

"Hey," says Cute Pharmacy Dude, greeting me. He's one of the few actual—not TV—people I see on a frequent basis.

He smiles through the pick-up window. The sun's shining and the sky is a cloudless blue. "Looks like it'll be a beautiful weekend."

"Yes, hopefully," I respond, handing him my insurance card.

"Have any big plans?"

Oh my goodness! Is he flirting with me?

"Going to my son's basketball games," I reply, batting my three eyelashes.

"Well, have a good one."

When I park in front of the grocery store, I take a quick look in the rearview mirror. Considering that I'm bald underneath my bandanna, pudgy, red-faced, and sweaty, it's safe to assume he wasn't putting the moves on me.

I've got to get out more.

~

Mom calls as soon as she gets the pathology report. "They didn't get clean margins."

"I'm sorry."

"Me, too." Her words are weighted down, in sharp contrast to her cheerful default mode. "The surgeon says the DCIS is more widespread than initially believed. And that it's fairly aggressive."

"What is he advising?"

"Well, I like this oncology surgeon so much better; I'm glad I left that other practice. But now I have to consider mastectomy. The doctor said he could do another lumpectomy, but there's the chance he still wouldn't get it all. So I have to make a decision. I'm going to spend some time thinking it over."

We'd hoped the first lumpectomy would achieve clear margins and could be followed up with radiation to rid her body of DCIS, a pretty straightforward treatment path. But once again, cancer acts sneaky and complicated. I hate this fricking disease!

~

I have good intentions to lead a healthier life, but the more I research known and suspected carcinogens, the more stressed

I feel. One news report warns that many body lotions and moisturizers contain estrogens, making them unsafe for cancer patients like myself. Another article cautions that grapefruit can interfere with the absorption of tamoxifen, one of the drugs used to prevent recurrence.

Experts disagree whether soy is helpful or harmful. Some warn that mega doses of vitamins can backfire, possibly undermining chemotherapy by artificially propping up your immune system.

How do I make healthy choices?

Too many items encountered on a daily basis are, or may be, carcinogenic.

Though I've managed to avoid tanning beds, asbestos, radon, etc., I've been exposed to BPA plastics, the lining of aluminum cans, char-grilled meats, sodium nitrate, alcohol, hair color, artificial sweeteners, parabens in beauty products, pesticides, radiation, sun exposure, second-hand smoke. Where will it end?

Has my life been a petri-dish for cancer?

Unless I move to a commune where we grow our own food, on an island with clean air and no water pollution, it's going to be impossible to avoid all carcinogens.

But I can do a better job of minimizing my exposure.

~

I start packing for a "girlfriends getaway" with Beth, redeeming some of our cancelled cruise credits. She's been dealing with tons of stress, too, and needs a break.

My phone rings; it's Beth. The last time she called, she'd told me to pack a plaid shirt and lumberjack boots, joking that if some loser guy was hitting on her, I should ditch my wig and pretend to be her rainbow lover. I'd scolded her not to stereotype, that most lesbians I knew had great style.

But this time, as soon as she says "Hello," I know something's wrong. "I'm sorry, Jo. But I can't go."

Divine Secret: Make positive changes and practice moderation.

Kudos for choosing a healthier lifestyle! But remember that it's okay to drink a glass of wine or eat a frosted cupcake every so often. Do a little research. Read labels. Check your grocery shelves; organic has gone mainstream!

"What's going on?"

"My dad's not getting better. Mom's asking me to stay here. She's never, ever done that."

"I totally understand. I'm sorry." I send up a prayer for Beth's father, a kind man with twinkling humor in his eyes and mercy in his heart.

When I get off the phone, I tell Ryan what's happened. That I'm going to cancel the trip.

"No, you should go," he insists. "Ask someone else."

"It wouldn't be the same." The cruise departs in a few days. I could invite another friend, but then I'd have to act cheerful and touristy, whereas I can be totally honest with Beth."

"Then go by yourself!" he urges. "You'd be crazy not to. Wouldn't you rather spend a few days by the pool instead of doing laundry and cooking dinner?"

"I'm worried about Mom."

"Worrying won't help anyone. You'll be back before she has surgery again."

Maybe he's right. After all, if that *Eat, Pray, Love* chick can spend three months traveling solo through Italy, India, and Indonesia, then surely I can spend three days lounging on a cruise deck.

Resources: Looking for healthy meal ideas? A few suggestions:

♦ Lisa Grey's *Pink Kitchen* cookbook collection (including volumes on soups, scones, and pestos) at pinkkitchen.info
♦ Leanne Ely's *Saving Dinner the Vegetarian Way* at savingdinner.com
♦ Kris Carr's cookbook *Crazy Sexy Diet: Eat Your Veggies, Ignite Your Spark, and Live Like You Mean It!*

My Version of *Eat, Pray, Love*

February 2008

I've always vacationed with family or close friends, but under these circumstances, the concept of a solo cruise actually appeals. I know plenty of people who could go in Beth's place, but there're only a few I'd really welcome. I need this time and space to mend my ragged emotions, not feel forced to act sociable and happy. Mary Lou, my other BFF in Texas, is dealing with family health issues, so she can't go. I know my closest local pals wouldn't be able to arrange child-care on short notice or swing a last-minute airline fare. An only child, I'm quite independent and not at all daunted by the idea of travelling alone.

So I pack up my bags and fly into the port city, where I catch the cruise line bus to the ship terminal. The people sitting nearby start chatting. They all have lovely, straight white teeth that look like Chiclets. The guy in the next row confides that they're all attending a cosmetic dentistry convention on board. *I'd better remember to floss between meals.*

After arriving at the terminal, I go through the check-in line, where a porter takes my suitcase. I keep a small carry-on with my swimsuit, medication, and cosmetics. Then I end up in a long, slow line that feels like a cattle call, where I amuse myself by people-watching.

Like a lot of things in life, reality never quite lives up to the fantasy. I remember the first time I went to Las Vegas. I'd expected the casinos to have an elegant, sophisticated vibe: men dressed like Frank Sinatra or James Bond, women wearing sparkly evening gowns, dripping in diamonds. Instead, I saw the unwashed masses in sneakers and stretch pants, frantically cramming nickels from plastic cups into slot machines.

Mom and Pop have taken some upscale cruises, where male passengers wear tuxedos to dinner, and every cabin has butler service. But looking around at my fellow vacationers—decked out in cut-off jeans, muscle t-shirts, and floral muumuus—I fear this ship may be the Wal-Mart of cruise lines.

Finally, I reach a second check-in counter. A female cruise line official looks at my passport and ticket. "You're staying in the cabin alone? There's no one travelling with you?"

"Yes, my friend had to cancel at the last minute."

"Oh, that's terrible. You couldn't find anyone else?"

Despite the Jimmy Buffett–style Muzak playing in the background, it feels less "Welcome to Paradise," more "Welcome to Loserville."

"I'm sure I *could* have found someone but I'm *choosing* to travel alone."

"Oh, okay," she replies with a forced smile, her eyes full of pity. She hands me back my passport. "I hope you enjoy your cruise."

Then I'm forced to stop for the mandatory pre-boarding photo, standing on a faux ship backdrop, complete with railing and a porthole.

"Where's everyone else?" asks the photographer.

"It's just me."

"Really? Oh, okay. Then smile."

I follow the line to the gangway and walk aboard the ship. My big suitcase sits outside my cabin; inside a bouquet of roses from Ryan awaits me. *Dang, I'm a lucky girl!*

I'm still unpacking when I hear an announcement over the P.A system: "Joanna Chapman, please come to the purser's desk."

I climb several flights of stairs to the deck with the atrium lobby and grand piano. At the desk, I hand the gentleman clad in a navy-blue jacket and brass nametag my cruise card and passport.

"Ms. Chapman, our records are showing you travelling alone. Is this correct?"

"Yes."

"So you don't have a companion booked with you? We can't leave port until all passengers are confirmed."

"My friend had to cancel," I reply through gritted teeth. "Yes, I'm travelling alone. There is no one else in my cabin."

"I'm sorry," he says.

Now I'm starting to get pissed off. I don't remember Elizabeth Gilbert, author of *Eat, Pray, Love*, being viewed as an object of pity as she crossed the globe.

I chose to come alone, so I'd have the freedom to read non-stop, sleep as much as I wanted, or never leave my lounge chair, without having to accommodate the wishes of anyone else. But I'm sure there are plenty of nice people, through no fault of their own, who have to travel alone if they want a vacation. Perhaps they are widowed or single and their friends are too broke to join them. Sure hope these cruise ships don't treat all their solo travelers like losers.

~

Leaning against the rail, I watch as we sail away from the port. Soothed by the rhythm of the waves, baptized by the salty spray, I feel contemplative, dedicating the next few days for reflection and inner healing. To come to terms with what's happened and with what my future may hold.

Wish I could see Cancerland fade away in my rearview mirror, but this is more rest stop than exit. I'm still facing reconstructive surgery, frequent checkups with Rock Star Surgeon and Dr. Point Guard, plus years of anti-hormonal medications.

Some aspects of my journey have been easier than anticipated, others tougher. Many days I was confused, fearful, and frustrated. Yet other times I was inspired to laugh out loud and felt love wrap around me like a fuzzy, hand-knitted shawl. There's no way I can repay my friends, family, and sister survivors.

But could I pay it forward? Would sharing my experiences help anyone?

Many years ago, my third grade teacher told me I had a gift for writing. Her compliment has stayed with me for decades. *But how could she tell?* It's not like anyone hands out Pulitzer Prizes to elementary school students. During college, one of my English professors predicted I'd write a book someday. He was probably imagining a scholarly tome about Emily Dickinson's poetry rather than boobs and foobs.

*Maybe I **could** write a book.*

Granted, it would be more literary Hamburger Helper than black truffle pâté. I might come across like an oversharing idiot. But what if my personal narrative helped others feel less confused, crazy, frightened, and alone?

Pulling a legal pad from my tote bag, I start jotting down notes. I never kept a diary when I was a teenager, perhaps afraid someone would read it, violating my privacy. Or possibly I preferred to ignore my tangled emotions rather than unravel them. It comes as a revelation now how soul-cleansing it feels to jot down my thoughts.

~

That afternoon, I schedule a hot stone massage at the spa. Before my appointment, I have to fill out paperwork. One question asks if I've had cancer in the past five years. I answer honestly. Batting my anxiety away, I sink into a plush chair and sip a cup of herbal tea, listening to New Age music and the bubbling of a tabletop rock fountain. A cheerful masseuse with a British accent calls my name and escorts me to a treatment room. She looks at my paperwork and frowns. "I'm not sure I can give you a massage. The aromatherapy oils are strong. They might activate your lymphatic system, causing the cancer to spread."

What the heck? If massage was risky, then why do so many oncology centers employ massage therapists? British Masseuse leaves to consult with her boss. I wait on the therapy table, moping. A spa treatment sounded like such a lovely idea.

"All right, my supervisor has given permission for the hot stone treatment," she says, closing the door behind her. "But to be safe, I'll use a mild oil and not massage you quite so vigorously."

Having warm rocks rubbed on my back is living dangerously? Really?

For the rest of this trip, I avoid the spa and seek my bliss poolside.

I dress up for dinner and go to the early show, where dancers in cheesy nautical outfits sing a pop medley. Arriving at the dining room, I discover an error; I've been assigned to the early seating, not the late. The maître d' apologizes and leads me to a temporary table for that evening.

I'm seated with a group of well-coiffed Texas socialites and their spouses. The women look stunning in their cocktail dresses and gold jewelry; the men sport Rolex watches. They're a friendly crowd, chatting as we peruse the menu.

"Tell us about yourself. What do you do?" asks the man sitting across from me. He's a husky guy with a thick mustache, silver hair, and a nice smile.

I pause for a nanosecond.

If I say stay-at-home mom, eyes will glaze over, my tablemates worried I'll share crockpot recipes and coupon clipping strategies.

But I watch Oprah. I've heard about The Secret, *the plan for charting your own destiny. I'm going to embrace the law of attraction, claim positive vibes from the universe, and make my dreams a reality!*

"I'm a writer."

"That sounds interesting," Mustache Man replies. "Do you work for a newspaper or magazine?"

"No. I'm actually, um, writing a book." No need to tell him that all I have so far is a few scribbled pages on a yellow legal-sized pad.

"What a coincidence!" He gestures toward the woman sitting to my right. "Katrina has a book coming out, too."

Ack, I'm such an idiot!

Gorgeous Author, a fine-featured, petite blonde, tells me about her book, a work of historical fiction based on family stories. *Just my luck!* Of all the people on the cruise ship—on the one night I work up the nerve to publicly profess I'm a writer—I end up beside a *bona fide* author for a major publishing house, with a release date and scheduled book-signing tour.

David Copperfield, please make me disappear!

The waiter brings our first course and refills everyone's beverage.

"Tell us about your book," says Gorgeous Author.

"It's a memoir, actually."

The conversation thuds to an awkward silence. They're all wondering why anyone would read a book about my life. But I've already discussed cancer once today and decline to bring it up again.

"Do you have a publication date?"

"No, I'm not finished yet."

Gorgeous Author gives me a gracious smile, even though I suspect she thinks I'm clueless. "Hang in there. It took me several years to finish my manuscript, then another year to find an agent."

Mustache Man starts up a conversation about cruise excursions. We discuss snorkeling adventures and shopping expeditions; I'm grateful for the change of topics.

There's an empty seat between me and Gorgeous Author. After the main course arrives, she invites me to move next to her. "Apparently, my husband's not coming," she explains. "He's battling cancer and gets tired easily."

Damn disease! Has to keep following me around.

"Gosh, I'm sorry." I meet her eyes, shaking my head. "I'm

recovering from cancer, too. The experience is the main focus of my book."

"It's pretty intense," she says, nodding. "Must have given you lots of material."

We start talking in cancer dialect—a language outsiders can't fully understand—sharing stories, comparing treatments, explaining how relationships were transformed. Before dessert is served, I bid my dinner companions farewell. As gracious as they've been, I'm hoping my tablemates for the rest of the cruise will be in perfect health, with no medical horror stories to share.

$\sim$

The next morning, I head to the pool deck. I avoid the crowded area near the steel drum band and select a lounge chair in a quiet area with a panoramic view. As soon as I settle in with my paperback and iPod, my floppy straw hat blows away, revealing my stubbly head. I lean over the railing and see it floating in the kiddie pool two decks below. Self-conscious about my near baldness, I retrieve it and sit back down.

Within minutes, my hat flies off again, so I chase it and move to a less windy location.

A woman in a nearby chair tries to start a chat. Her husband won't leave the casino and she's feeling bored. I don't want to be rude, but I don't really want to talk. So after exchanging a few pleasantries, I put in my earphones and bury my nose in the latest Carl Hiaasen book. I select the Red Hot Chili Peppers on my iPod, listening as the mournful wails of Anthony Kiedis echo the lingering wistfulness in my heart. Although the cruise line works hard to promote a festive atmosphere, with poolside conga lines, belly-flop contests, and upbeat music, I'm drawn to the quieter spots, where I can accommodate my melancholy.

I remember being surprised shortly after my diagnosis when a Pink Sister confessed that, nearly a year after chemo, she still felt depressed and couldn't enjoy life like before. At the time I didn't understand. *Wasn't she supposed to bounce back to "normal" by then?* Now I comprehend how cancer leaves you with a sense of loss. Not just about body parts, or hair, but your perception of invincibility, the belief that you are calling the shots in life.

~

That night at the early seating for dinner, I meet my tablemates: three women from a small town in East Texas and two flamingly gay men from Houston.

The ladies, with the first names of country singers—Loretta, Patty, and Reba—tighten their lips when Dennis, a male nurse, and his partner, Roger, tell us they are celebrating their five-year anniversary. *Really, a gay interior decorator and a nurse? Could they be making this up?*

Dennis hands Roger a small box. "Open it."

Inside is a thick silver link bracelet.

"Wow, Dennis. It's beautiful," Roger beams.

"I have one that matches," Dennis explains, holding out his arm.

"Congratulations!" I say.

The Country Music Trio close rank, rolling their eyes, and carrying on a private conversation. I, on the other hand, find the gay couple funny and personable, and laugh while they engage in some good-natured domestic squabbling.

"I can't believe you picked out such a great bracelet on your own," Roger adds.

"What, did you think I'd get you something tacky?"

Roger shrugs his shoulders and gives me a grin. "You should have seen the apartment he was living in when we met! Absolutely atrocious."

After the entrée, our waiter prepares Cherries Jubilee tableside, pouring liquor over fruit, then igniting it. Now our table is even more flaming.

~

I spend the next day at a private beach resort outfitted with comfy lounge chairs, umbrellas, snorkel gear, a lunch buffet, and an open bar. The sky is bright robin's egg blue, dotted with one or two white cottony clouds. The water is turquoise, so clear you can see the bottom. Waiters walk around the white sand beach, offering sodas or margaritas. As I listen to the piped-in music, a mash-up of Latino vocalists and classic rock guitar riffs, my mood is cheerful, not glum.

Ryan was right. This does beat laundry and grocery shopping!

Soaking up the warm rays of the sun, my thoughts turn inward. I mentally tabulate reasons to be grateful. My cancer was discovered at an early stage. Odds are very good it will never return. I have a supportive circle of friends and family. Our family has health insurance and enough money to pay the bills.

I wish all my Pink Sisters could have as much support. In a just world, cancer would afflict only bad people, like pedophiles and serial killers. Not little kids or kind, good-hearted people. I hate that some survivors face unfavorable statistics and will have to continue treatment for the rest of their lives.

I'm not going to take this second chance for granted.

~

Later that afternoon, the excursion bus takes us back to the cruise terminal for shopping. Inspired by my tablemates, I buy two turquoise bracelets, one for me, one for Beth, even though I love her in a platonic, not Sapphic, way. I find a small wooden marlin for Alex, who's an avid fisherman, and onyx pyramids for Nick and Ryan, both intrigued by ancient cultures. For Larissa, the Empress of Dress-up, I select a white pleated folk dress with embroidery.

Back on the ship, I head to an upper deck, to watch the spectacular view as we sail away. As we head to open sea, the water is eerily flat like textured glass, while the sky fills with a diffuse glow, golden rays painted on the clouds. The vista reminds me of a Thomas Kinkade painting, almost too beautiful and serene to be real.

Awed by nature, I feel the presence and permanence of God. As if on cue, the Beatles' hit "Let it Be" echoes through the sound system. A sense of peace enfolds me, chasing away my neurotic fears. Maybe that *Eat, Pray, Love* chick found her spiritual enlightenment scrubbing floors in India. I'll look for mine at sunset on the cruise deck.

The song ends, and the music shifts to the "Cupid Shuffle." Two dozen members of an extended family are on board to celebrate both a wedding and a golden anniversary. The group fills the dance floor, the bride resplendent in a satin gown with seed pearls and lace, her groom clad in a white tuxedo. They are surrounded by bridesmaids in shiny taffeta dresses, each one a different rainbow color. Men in sherbet-colored suits kick and turn to the music. My heart swells as I watch the group, united in rhythm and love.

My time for renewal and reflection has been a luxury. Though I've met friendly people aboard, I've cherished the time spent alone to think about my future. And reflect on what type of legacy I want to leave.

Maybe one of the highest callings in life is to be kind. But not a syrupy Southern niceness. Something more substantial. I vow to be mindful of my interactions, more tolerant of my husband's quirks, less quick to take offense. To show more patience with my children, even on the days when they seem more like *Rosemary's Babies* than my own. To become a better, more considerate friend. To act gracious even to really annoying people.

On the last evening of the cruise, while browsing through the photo gallery, I'm struck by the portrait of a couple. The woman is wearing a long red dress, but the inch or two of bristly jagged hair, forced smile, and vacant expression give her away as a survivor. Either that or she lost a fight with a weed whacker. I don't know anything about her or her situation, but I wish I could give her some "Dark Cherry" lipstick, sparkly earrings, and a hug.

In a show of solidarity with the sad-eyed woman, to let her know she's not alone, I decide to go to dinner without my wig. I rub hair paste into my fuzzy baby-chick hair, making it as spiky and vertical as possible. Surprisingly, I do not feel embarrassed by this look; I feel liberated, healthy, and whole. Granted, my new coiffure is not exactly attractive, but I'm happy to see my own hair growing back. The woman in the picture and I never speak, but we make eye contact across the dining room. I smile at her, and she smiles back.

~

The travel home from vacation is always such a buzz kill. After spending a few great days of rest and relaxation, it seems I'm always dealing with cancelled airline flights and endless lines, only to arrive home to a fridge with outdated milk and suitcases stuffed with dirty laundry.

Disembarking from a cruise has a unique unpleasantness. First, the restaurants are madhouses because breakfast service stops around 7 a.m. Then, you have to leave your cabin and cool your heels sitting, bleary-eyed, in the auditorium or one of the ship's lounges until your deck number is called.

After exiting the ship, I walk outside the port terminal to one of the airport shuttle buses. My flight doesn't leave for several hours, so I should have plenty of time to check in and browse the airport bookstore before boarding.

Except that my bus isn't going anywhere.

After thirty minutes, I leave my seat to talk to the driver. "What's the deal? The bus is pretty full. Why aren't we leaving?"

"I have to wait for all the other buses. We leave at the same time."

"That doesn't make sense! There are another half-dozen buses here. Some people have a very short window to catch their flight and others have nearly all day."

She looks at me and shrugs.

I walk back to my seat and take some deep, calming breaths.

Kindness, I remind myself. My new goal in life. I eat a bag of peanut M&Ms, fretting that I probably won't have time for lunch in the airport before my flight.

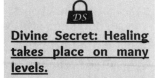

Divine Secret: Healing takes place on many levels.

Your body will recuperate, but your spirit needs time to recover, too. Give yourself permission to deal with sad, angry, and scared feelings, but try to find a way to move forward. Look for opportunities to reflect on your cancer journey and how it has changed you. Rest, renew, recharge.

When the bus driver finally pulls out of the cruise terminal parking lot, I'm not the only cranky passenger.

Some of the dentists from the on-board conference are checking their watches. But since they are all frowning, I can't admire their nice teeth.

As we near the airport, the passengers start asking which terminal they need.

"Uh, A?" says Ditzy Bus Driver. "Or maybe B?"

One of the dentists is flying home on a regional jet and totally confused about where to go for his code/share flight. Since the bus driver can't offer a definitive answer, I text Ryan.

"C," I tell the dentist.

I get off at the next terminal stop, along with a cluster of other cruise passengers. We wait on the sidewalk while Ditzy Bus Driver unloads suitcases from the luggage compartment. Once there are no more suitcases to unload on this side, she goes to the other side of the bus and carries more bags to the sidewalk. I'm standing there, watching everyone else get their suitcases, and still waiting for mine when the bus starts to drive away.

"Stop! Stop!" I yell, flailing my arms like a crazy lady. "My suitcase!"

The bus driver slams on the brakes and looks annoyed. She retrieves my bag and places it on the sidewalk in a grudging manner, without any apology.

"Hey, lady!" I yell, as she turns and walks back to the bus. "You might want to figure out which airlines fly out of which terminals. Might be good to know..."

She drives away.

My vow of perpetual kindness? What can I say? I'm a work-in-progress.

Resources: Retreats for survivors:

♦ Book a cabin on one of the "Thrivers" cruises hosted by breastcancerwellness.org

♦ Learn to fish during a free (application required) 2.5 day retreat with castingforrecovery.org

♦ Enjoy a free (application required) weeklong beach stay at littlepinkhousesofhope.org

---

Short on money or vacation days?

Consider an afternoon at a botanical garden. Or a do-it-yourself home spa day. Or a budget-friendly spiritual retreat. The key is to find something restorative, where you have time to reflect and recharge, to look back but to also look forward.

Resource: Book

Woman's Comfort Book: A Self-Nurturing Guide for Restoring Balance in Your Life, by Jennifer Louden

More Like a Bad Hair Year

Back home, I have good intentions to move forward, but keep getting stuck in emotional quicksand. I remember when one Pink Sister posted on a survivorship bulletin board that on the way home from the hospital, she stopped at Target to do a little shopping!

To her, breast cancer was not a big deal.

Naturally, her insensitive comment morphed into a running joke.

Maybe she really felt that way. But I suspect the bitter after-taste of cancer caught up with her eventually. From what I've heard, getting to the "new normal" is a process with steps forward and back. Most Pink Sisters juggle a multitude of emotions: grief over physical and emotional losses, gratitude for being alive, anger over what cancer has stolen, empathy for sister survivors, and a lingering fear of recurrence.

Though I wrestle with these same emotions, I resolve to "get busy living." I'll volunteer at Larissa's school, polish my resume, and make plans for the future.

But as the weeks go by, I'm body-slammed with more bad news.

Since Mom's breast MRI and pathology report shows extensive and aggressive DCIS, with her doctor's advice, she decides on a mastectomy.

Beth's older brother dies of Stage IV kidney cancer. Her father's health continues to decline.

Patrick Swayze is diagnosed with pancreatic cancer.

I've never met the hunky dancer/actor, yet his news is the proverbial last straw. I hide in my bedroom, shades drawn, watching *Dirty Dancing* and *Ghost. Nobody puts Johnny Castle in the corner!*

The bad feelings aren't over, not by a long shot.

~

Ryan and the kids start talking about getting another dog. But I'm content having only one, a sweet but yappy miniature dachshund.

"Mom, he only barks because he's lonely," says Alex.

"He'd be happier with a friend," says Ryan. "And then the neighbors would be less annoyed."

"Please, Mommy," adds Larissa.

After everything that's happened lately, our family could really use a little fun, something joyful to anticipate, so I agree. I look at local animal shelter websites and fill out an adoption application.

A few days later, several women from the animal shelter bring Rover, a medium size mix breed with big brown eyes, over for a home visit. They explain that he was a very shy stray who survived on stolen cat food and that it had taken a long time before he would get close to them.

Fido immediately warms up to our guest and before you know it, the two are frolicking together in the back yard. After playing awhile, Rover comes up to the deck and puts his head in my lap, gazing up at me.

Okay, I'm in love. This dog now has a family.

Unfortunately, one of the women is experiencing separation anxiety at the thought of leaving her canine companion behind.

Foster Dog Mom corners me on the deck. "What are you going to feed him? There's a special brand he likes but you can only get it by mail-order."

Before I can answer, she asks another question, "Where is he going to sleep? He prefers his master's bed."

"Thanks for telling me," I smile and nod as the other woman tries to get Foster Dog Mom to leave.

"Look," she says, peeling Foster Dog Mom's fingers from the deck railing. "He's happy. He'll be fine."

"Yes," I say. "He fits in perfectly with our family."

~

Divine Secrets: Survivorship is a process.

In recent years, studies have demonstrated a need for survivorship services—counseling, physical therapy, information about side effects—that continue after a cancer patient finishes active treatment. Many nurse navigators now schedule follow-up appointments to help with this transition.

Getting dressed for yet another appointment with Rock Star Surgeon, I realize why some old people yammer incessantly about health issues. It's because encounters for medical care may be the bulk of their social interactions. I've spent more time in the past six months chatting with doctors, nurses, and Cute Pharmacy Dude than my friends.

But at least today's appointment has forced me out of pajamas. I glance in the mirror, and wince at my reflection. I'd look more attractive with the wig, but wearing it reminds me of being a patient. I'm happy to have some hair, even if it's barely more than stubble. I spike it up with gel then put on lipstick and dangling earrings to avoid the androgynous Peter Pan look.

Slipping out of my bathrobe, I start to dress. But I can't find the clone! I'm certain I left it on the bathroom counter. Not there. I look inside the closet and search the dresser drawers. The clock is ticking; I have to leave soon. Feeling desperate, about to stuff my bra with a pair of socks, I spot Larissa pushing her doll carriage. I peek inside. She's swaddled my clone in a hand towel like an alien baby. I grab it and stuff it in my bra while she wails.

"Sorry, sweetie. But Mommy's booby is not a toy."

~

I tell Rock Star Surgeon about my mom's diagnosis. He knows I've been considering a prophylactic mastectomy.

"Really? Who's her surgeon?" he asks.

"Not anyone here. She lives several hours away, in the mountains."

"I want you to have BRCA testing done. The results will show whether you have any known genetic risk for breast or ovarian cancer," he explains. "If you know your true risk, you can make an informed decision."

"Okay." I cross my arms and fidget on the crinkly exam table paper. "I may still want my breast removed, regardless of test results."

Rock Star Surgeon sighs. I must be one of his most exasperating patients.

"Sometimes people feel that way at first. But remember, if I take it off, I can't put it back on. I don't want you to have any regrets or make a hasty decision."

~

Within a month, I've gone from the G.I. Jane buzz to the short, coarse curls some of my Pink Sisters have dubbed "sheep's ass hair." But I think it makes me look like a Chia Pet. As a child, my hair was blonde, but it darkened over the years. At the moment, it's an unflattering mix of gray and dark brown, so I decide to color it at home, aiming for a nice strawberry blonde. Alas, my results in no way resemble the model on the package.

"Wow, Mom, your hair's really orange!" Alex says.

He's right. I look like Ronald McDonald's evil twin.

"Mommy has orange hair, Mommy has orange hair," Larissa sings.

Divine Secret: Your hair will grow back, but not overnight.

It takes an agonizingly long time, but your hair will probably return to your natural texture and color. However—trust me on this—leave the coloring to salon professionals!

"Thanks, guys, for the encouragement."

Later that night, Ryan makes a gentle suggestion. "Honey, why don't you go to a salon? Don't worry about the money."

Obviously, my hair is a total disaster.

Renovation:

My Extreme Cancer Makeover

Digging Up Family Skeletons

Spring 2008

Mom helped us so much during my surgeries and chemo. When she has her mastectomy, I feel guilty that I can't stay at her house for an extended period. Ryan's job requires a lot of travel; I can't leave the kids for long. But I arrange to make a short overnight trip to visit after her surgery.

My folks are both retired, with lots of supportive friends willing to drop off dinner. Nevertheless, I make a few meals—amazing what you can do with a can of soup and some bread crumbs!—and pack them in a cooler for the drive to the mountains.

I'm in the car, on my way, when my cell phone rings. It's Mom.

"How are you feeling?"

"Not great." Her words are slurred.

"I'll be there soon."

"Joanna, could you please stop at the drugstore? There's something I need."

My poor mother! She's in the hospital, for Pete's sake, and she's not getting what she needs! Is she in pain? Nauseated from the anesthesia? I'm ready to storm the nurses station like Shirley MacLaine in *Terms of Endearment.*

"Of course. What can I get you?"

"I really need some pink lip gloss."
It's a make-up emergency.
She's going to be just fine.

~

A few days later, there's a thick manila envelope in my mail-box, a questionnaire to fill out before meeting with the genetics counselor.

I wade through hundreds of questions about my health and the medical history of my biological parents, siblings, grand-parents, great-grandparents, aunts, uncles, and cousins.

Part of the form is easy to fill out, because I have no siblings. My list of biological maternal relatives is fairly small, with one aunt, one uncle, one female cousin, and two male cousins. Though there's been high blood pressure and diabetes on this side of my family tree, there's no prior family history of cancer.

However, the paternal side of my family is a Pandora's box I don't want to open. I close my eyes and rub my temples, trying to ward off an impending migraine. My headaches have gotten worse since my recent medication change from tamoxifen to an aromatase inhibitor. I make a mental note to ask Dr. Point Guard and my neurologist about this.

I stare at the form, pen in mid-air. I'm tempted to claim that I have no information. Maybe if half my family medical history is missing, my insurance would be more inclined to pay for testing. But I'm too honest for that. Also, it's hard to claim ignorance in the age of Google.

Though handsome and intelligent, my late biological father was a selfish, troubled man, with little interest in parenting. I've had virtually no contact with that side of my family for the past 30 years. The last communication I received was in 2002, a copy of my father's obituary and a photo of my uncle Robert's two adolescent daughters, Hannah and Ashley, my biological cousins.

I cried a bit over the clipping, not out of grief, but for the sense of lost possibility. Never in my childhood was I doted upon as a "Daddy's Girl." If I'd had a loving father, would I have turned out to be a sweeter, less brittle person?

The whole nature versus nurture conundrum perplexes me.

Staring into the mirror, I don't see much physical resemblance to my father, his brother, or my paternal grandparents, all tall and slender, some with black hair, others with red. My DNA contains some of their genetic material, but I don't look anything like them.

Studying my reflection, I note that I have neither their high cheekbones nor their piercing eyes.

But what's that on my upper lip?

Moving closer to the mirror, I confirm my suspicions. A brown mustache hair!

Ack! I grab the tweezers.

I've joked about feeling like a hollow chocolate Easter bunny after having so many internal parts removed. *But without any estrogen or many female organs left, could I be turning into a dude?* The only upside would be if chosen for *Dancing with the Stars*, I'd be paired with nice Karina Smirnoff rather than bossy Maksim Chmerkovskiy. And maybe I'd look good in a spray tan and sequins.

I glance at the clock, realizing the kids will be home soon, so I put away the family history medical forms. I didn't carry Larissa in my womb, but my love for her is as fierce as for my sons. Still, I can't deny certain qualities—her compassion, gracefulness, innate sense of direction—that weren't inherited from Ryan or me. She's starting to ask questions about her first months in China, trying to understand the different definitions of family.

I have several friends who were adopted as babies and express no desire to search for biological relatives. They say the people who raised them are their family. I have the same perspective. Families are bonded more by love than by blood. When I first met Pop, I was already grown and married, a little skeptical and unwilling to invest much emotional energy in getting to know him. But over the years, we've grown to love each other like most dads and daughters.

Still, there are eerie connections sometimes with biological relatives. I dig out the photo of my uncle's daughters from a box in my closet. Their resemblance to my paternal second cousin, Linda, and me as teenagers is uncanny. Ashley, long and lanky, has Linda's prominent brow and sharp features, like the rest of the clan. Hannah is shorter and rounded, with softer features, like me. In the letter, my uncle describes his daughters as horse-lovers and avid readers, traits we share.

I wonder how things might have been different. Would I have been the fun older cousin who hosted sleepovers and went to their horse shows? I'll never know; some bridges are too difficult to cross.

I was a child of the 70s, a time when divorces seemed much less congenial than they do today. Weekend visitation meetings with the non-custodial parents were arranged like ransom drops, the kids and their suitcases exchanged at a fast-food restaurant or other neutral location.

After each of her daughters' divorces, my maternal grandmother took a pair of scissors to her photo collection, snipping out images of her ex-sons-in-law, leaving portraits of brides walking solo down the aisle, holding onto disembodied arms. In a similar way, I've chosen to erase certain people from my life.

Yet, because of biology, family health history matters. I need to contact my uncle, my father's younger brother. Taking a deep breath, I google Robert's full name and profession, skimming through several articles referencing his business and hobbies.

Then, staring at the screen, I gasp.

He's dead.

Passed away a few years ago.

From Stage IV *colon cancer*.

Still young, only in his mid-50s.

I shiver, as if I've stumbled into a walk-in freezer. When I was first diagnosed, I knew of no family members with cancer. But now there are three.

Mom.

My uncle.

Me.

~

Within a day or two, I'm able to track down Robert's business partner, who then puts me in touch with Penny, his widow.

I feel awkward calling her; I only met her once, when I was in college. But I do need to ask her some questions.

To my relief, she is pleasant and open.

"It's been years, but I'm glad to hear from you, Joanna," she says. "Although I'm sorry about the circumstances. About your cancer."

"Thanks. And I'm sorry for your loss, Penny."

"It was a total surprise. The doctors thought he had it beat, but it recurred."

We are both silent for a minute, thinking of how much we hate cancer.

"Are you aware of any family history?" I ask.

"None whatsoever. Cancer wasn't even on our radar."

Before ending our conversation, she invites me to visit whenever I'm in the area. Says her girls would enjoy meeting me. But I don't want to disturb ghosts from the past. I'm sure these biological cousins are delightful young women. But I have no real connection with them; just some shared cytoplasm. Who your true family is involves much more than DNA.

Divine Secret: Consider genetic testing to find out your inherited risk of cancer.

Not everyone with a family history of breast cancer wants genetic testing, but it can help you better understand your risk. You can be more proactive in monitoring your health and share what you've learned with other family members.

<u>Resources: Learn more about hereditary breast cancers:</u>

Myriad Labs performs genetic testing for BRCA1 and BRCA2 and now offers testing for other hereditary cancers, such as colorectal and melanoma. Talk to your doctor and read more at <u>myriad.com</u>. FORCE, Facing Our Risk of Cancer Empowered, is a nonprofit designed to help individuals and families affected by hereditary breast cancer. Their website <u>facingourrisk.org</u> offers education and support as well as an annual conference.

Last Hope for Making Major Lemonade

As the weather warms and the first flowers bloom, Ryan and I travel several hours to consult with another plastic surgeon. I'm still hoping to finagle that free tummy-tuck. Working at a top-notch university and medical center, Renowned Plastic Surgeon is one of the few doctors in our state who performs DIEP (Deep Inferior Epigastric Perforator), the complex and delicate procedure to create "foobs" from abdominal tissue without compromising any muscle.

As Ryan and I walk through the beautiful, leafy campus, I cross my fingers. The patient photos on the doctor's website are impressive. Yes, I'm obsessing over reconstruction, but I'm still trying so hard to squeeze a little lemonade out of this whole sour experience.

After a few minutes in the exam room, Renowned Plastic Surgeon has discouraging news. "You don't have enough excess tissue for a bilateral operation."

The hopeful smile slides right off my face.

Hard to believe, with my Buddha belly!

"I'd recommend a DIEP reconstruction on the right side, with a reduction and lift of your natural left breast for symmetry."

Ryan nods in agreement. *What does he know?*

"I won't know for certain whether I can do the DIEP until we're in the operating room."

Since the procedure involves microsurgical grafting of tiny blood vessels, eligibility depends on my anatomy. Renowned Plastic Surgeon warns me there's a 40% chance he'll have to do a TRAM procedure instead, harvesting muscle, with an increased risk of permanent side effects. Either way, there'd be a lengthy hospital stay and challenging recovery. My Pink Sisters who've had DIEP seem delighted with their results, but I dread another long hospitalization. I'm not keen on a reduction and lift of my remaining breast, either, because the degree of symmetry achieved varies widely. Also, I'm awaiting my BRCA results and considering a prophylactic mastectomy.

"Why don't you think it over?" Renowned Plastic Surgeon bids us goodbye. "Call my nurse if you want to schedule an additional consultation."

Ryan reaches for my hand as we walk to the parking garage. "Did you like him?" he asks.

"Yeah, the doctor seems great. But I'm not sure I want a single-sided DIEP."

Ryan sighs. "I think he gave you a good option. DIEP on the right, reduction and lift on the left."

"Glad you both agree." Sarcasm creeps into my voice.

"What he said made sense. Why not keep the natural one?"

Ryan's trying to be supportive, so I shouldn't get snippy. I explain that I'll be the one looking in the mirror, feeling for lumps, returning for life-long follow-up appointments, wrestling with anxiety. Deep inside my gut, I don't think Renowned Plastic Surgeon's recommendation is the path I want to take.

Divine Secret: Investigate all reconstruction options.

Find a surgeon specializing in reconstructive surgery, because it's nothing like a standard breast augmentation. Ask to see photos. Keep in mind that many surgeons prefer one procedure over the others, so look into all your options. There are pros and cons to each choice. Figure out what's best for you.

Spotting our car, Ryan clicks the remote. We get inside and buckle our seatbelts.

"Why can't you just follow the doctor's advice?"

"It's my body," I retort, slamming the door. "Shouldn't I get the final vote?"

Sweating for the Cure

Despite trying to keep up a positive attitude, I continue struggling with post-treatment doldrums. *How come nobody warns you that the time **after** cancer is unexpectedly tough?* The concept seems counter-intuitive. But in the post-treatment months, strong waves of emotion can surge and knock you down. You may feel adrift on a lonely sea, as interactions with your medical team subside.

Ryan is starting to lose patience with me. He comes into the bedroom while I'm getting dressed. "You need to stop spending so much time on that pink website."

"No, it really helps me."

"Doesn't seem that way to me," he complains. "You need to find something productive to do. Stop moping all the time. Forget about cancer."

"Oh, really? I'm supposed to forget about cancer?" I jerk my pajama top open. "Exactly how am I supposed to do that? When I have to look in the mirror each day?"

"Shouldn't you be moving on? Instead of hiding out in the bedroom?"

"But I can't just move on. Mom's still dealing with cancer. My hair's an ugly mess and will be for months. I need several reconstructive surgeries. Maybe *then* I can stop moping about cancer!"

"Fine," he says, walking out of the bedroom. "Suit yourself."

Moving past cancer is not a linear, deadline-oriented process. Some days it feels like two steps forward, three steps back. He just doesn't get it.

~

After Mom recovers from the mastectomy, her plastic surgeon inserts an expander where her breast once was to stretch her skin and muscle. Eventually he'll swap it out for an implant. But she develops a painful seroma—a collection of fluid at the surgical site—that a nurse has to drain with a needle. *Guess those icky surgical drains aren't such a bad idea after all!*

~

At the computer, I check the *YSC* message board, my heart sinking as I notice that another name has been added to the remembrance board. I have not met these ladies in person. Perhaps I knew only their first names or user IDs—MamaCath, Shabby, Dr. Melinda—but they shared their hearts. I'm in awe of how brave and generous they were, embracing frightened newcomers to this awful sorority despite their own dark struggles. After a silent prayer, I blink the tears away and open my e-mail.

My mailbox is stuffed full, mostly with spam. As I delete unwanted messages, I come across one that makes me furious. Bossy PTO Mom has sent an e-mail to Nick's teacher, practically accusing me of fraud! A week or two ago, I'd signed a form confirming my intent to participate in a year-long gift card fundraiser, so that Nick could enter a contest to win an iPod. But when I tried to register on the website, most of the stores were located in Wisconsin or Minnesota, so I assumed I had the wrong URL and made a mental note to follow up. Preoccupied with other stuff, I forgot about it.

My fingers type in a flurry, composing a snarky response stating that I'm so sorry for missing the deadline but I've been preoccupied with *cancer*. That my mom is recovering from *cancer* surgery and that I'm barely past my own *cancer* experience. Furthermore, that our family already owns several iPods and that I would *never* scam the school!

My hand is poised over the "send" key. I hesitate, then hit "delete." I barely know Bossy PTO Mom. She's probably unaware that I've been sucked into the swirly pink vortex. Still, I've been a long-time school volunteer. I've bought cookie dough, coupon books, and gift wrap. Bid on silent auction baskets. Worked the cakewalk at school carnivals. Assisted with holiday parties and field trips. I wish she'd contacted me first instead of assuming the worst.

This is my wake-up call. I've been living in a bubble. My life may have been turned upside down by cancer, but the world has kept on spinning.

I guess that, unlike Visa or Mastercard, the Cancer Card isn't accepted everywhere.

> **Resource: Get an authentic cancer card!**
>
> You can actually apply for a "Stupid Cancer" Visa Platinum card through stupidcancer.org, a nonprofit organization supporting young adults diagnosed with any type of cancer before age 40.

~

A few weeks later, at a breast cancer awareness event with Larissa's Brownie troop, I spot Kathleen, Dr. Gravitas, and their youngest daughter.

"Hi, Joanna," says Kathleen. "I didn't realize you were going to chaperone today."

"Yeah," I say, out of earshot of the girls. "What was I thinking?" I trade wry glances with Dr. Gravitas, who'd talked me through my Stage IV scare. "I've had about all the awareness I can stand."

They laugh, and then I accompany the girls to a craft table, where they make sparkly pink bookmarks. After they finish, our Brownie troop moves to the next station, where they poke a fake, plastic demo breast, feeling for lumps. I plaster a smile on my face, even though I cringe inside.

∿

Buoyed by Liz's offer to run with me in the upcoming Komen "Race for the Cure," I continue exercising at the YMCA on a regular basis, listening to a motivational playlist through my earphones. I jog on the treadmill until I get winded, then I switch to walking.

One day, I run (okay, jog) on the treadmill for an entire mile! Elated, caught up in the moment, I throw my hands in the air and imitate Sylvester Stallone's *Rocky* victory dance. Uh-oh…I realize I'm at the Y, not the steps in Philly. People on the Lifecycles are staring at me.

But who cares? I did it!

∿

A few weeks later, in May 2008, Liz, Hannah, Winona, Alex, and Nick join me in my first race. I jog the entire way, huffing and puffing, encouraged by crowds holding pink balloons and waving pom-poms. Some people walk faster than I can jog, but that's okay. I cross the finish line!

Ryan and Larissa wait for me at the end, along with Liz's husband and their two daughters.

"Good job, honey!"

"Yay for Mommy!"

Our group reconvenes for photos and high-fives. An announcement asks all survivors to meet at the Survivor Tent, where we're handed a pink carnation for every year

Divine Secret: Celebrate your survivorship.

Spend time with friends while helping in the fight against breast cancer. Participating in a race or walk might not be your thing, but you can donate to a team. Attend a silent auction or fundraising ball. Volunteer at your local hospital. Lobby your elected officials to increase research funds and restrict carcinogens.

since diagnosis. As music plays, we walk in procession to the
stage. I'm holding only one flower, but feel encouraged by the
women carrying huge bouquets. I think of my mother's diagnosis so soon after mine. When I look at the crowd, many of
them wearing a "Running in Memory of" sign, my throat tightens as I think about the loved ones who are no longer here.

Update: A Shout-Out to Nancy Brinker, founder of Susan G. Komen for the Cure

Over recent years, many have lobbed criticism at the Komen organization, perhaps some merited, some not. But I want to send a
little love to fellow survivor Nancy Brinker, the visionary and force
of nature who has transformed the battle against breast cancer,
using her talents as a fundraiser, spokesperson, and organizer. Her
efforts have raised awareness of breast cancer, funded research,
and provided health screenings to underserved populations.

We orbit in completely different social stratospheres. Nancy B.
inhabits the world of Neiman-Marcus, polo ponies, Limoges china,
and Baccarat crystal, while I'm more at home with Stein-mart
clearance racks, mini-golf, and microwave-safe dishes. Yet when
it comes to breast cancer, you could say that Nancy Brinker is my
"sista from another vista." Our stories resonate with many of the
same "aha" moments, such as when you realize that you must be
your own advocate. Or that you don't have to allow doctors to treat
you in a condescending, paternalistic way.

I can understand why people are unhappy at times with the Komen
organization. Granted, Komen has made missteps and taken
some PR hits over the years. A Pink Bucket of Fried Chicken for
the Cure? I mean, really? What's next, Chocolate-Glazed Donuts
for the Cure? Pork Rinds for the Cure?

But I'd like to ask everyone jumping on the anti-Komen bandwagon: What would living with breast cancer be like without Nancy
Brinker? Imagine a remake of It's a Wonderful Life, but instead
of the fictional George Bailey, the story revolved around Komen's
founder.

Would the words "breast" and "cancer" still be spoken in whispers
as if they were vulgarities? Would women in developing countries

have anywhere to turn for assistance? Would patients be expected to do what the doctor ordered, without question? Would women understand the importance of scheduling mammograms and checking out suspicious lumps?

So I urge you to remember the words of Clarence, the apprentice angel shadowing George Bailey: "Strange, isn't it? Each (wo)man's life touches so many other lives. When (s)he isn't around, (s)he leaves an awful hole, doesn't (s)he?"

Nancy Brinker, thanks for your efforts in the fight against breast cancer.

Shopping for a Second Honeymoon

Summer 2008

The past 12 months have been difficult, but I've reached the one-year mark since my diagnosis. The kids are out of school, so I take them to the pool, drive to sports camps, and arrange play dates for Larissa. I still spend too much time as a recluse, wasting hours caught up in my imaginary friendships with TV personalities. I need to hug Oprah goodbye, help Kendra clean up her room, and gently break the news to Holly that Hef is never, ever going to marry her.

One thing that elevates my mood, though, is planning an upcoming trip. To celebrate our 20th anniversary, Ryan and I are taking a cruise. My husband's not perfect—he's hard-wired with a time limit for empathetic listening—and neither am I, but he's been more princely than froggy throughout this ordeal.

So we're going to invest in making some great memories. The trip is definitely a splurge, a stretch to our budget, but the juxtaposition of happy/sad occasions—going on a trip/dealing with cancer—makes the joyous times even more jubilant. As those TV commercials pronounce, great experiences shared together are priceless.

I pick up the brochure, admiring the crystalline waters, exotic ports, and happy couples dressed in cocktail attire. Ryan and I share a love of travel and always have a great time on vacation.

We've stuck together for two decades; maybe it's time to bring back the spark. A European vacation is pricey, but I joke with Ryan that it's still cheaper than paying a divorce lawyer and splitting the 401(k). We've been vigilant about saving for retirement and college, but have gained a new appreciation for living in the moment, because everyone's days are numbered.

To show Ryan my love and appreciation, I plan to surprise him with a renewal of our wedding vows while on the cruise. To keep it a secret, I have the cruise line send the information to Mom's address.

Shopping for an appropriate dress for this special occasion is a challenge. Although some Pink Sisters may have the body type to wear a strapless dress, I do not. To accommodate my natural breast and the clone, I can't wear anything designed to show cleavage or with too large an arm hole. I'm flummoxed over what to wear for a vow renewal ceremony. Ryan and I did the whole '80s wedding thing. My dropped-waist satin gown had huge puffy sleeves, a full petticoat, and a lace-embellished train. At age 45, I'd feel silly wearing anything that looks too bridal, so nothing too poufy or floor-length. Also, the ceremony is just for the two of us, not a fancy reception with friends and family. But it is fun to browse in a shop or two. I've joked with Mom that I was deprived by being raised Protestant; I missed out on the lovely First Communion dresses and Bat Mitzvah party attire my friends enjoyed.

Divine Secret: Be patient and find your perfect special occasion dress.

You may want a dress to cover scars on your chest and under your armpit. Or maybe you're looking for a loosely fitted style to help disguise asymmetry. It may take some time, but don't stop shopping until you find something that makes you feel great. Think outside the box. Consider buying a larger sized dress with more bodice fabric that can be tailored to fit you just right. If your budget is tight, check out upscale consignment stores, which often have beautiful, barely worn cocktail dresses and evening gowns.

Divine Secret: Cancer can't stop you from being a beautiful bride.

Don't let cancer ruin your plans. You'll be gorgeous walking down the aisle. Talk to your bridal store consultant before you go in for an appointment. They can show you wedding dresses where adding sleeves or raising the neckline is an option. "Say Yes to the Dress" has some great episodes featuring brides battling cancer.

Yet I also want to avoid that whole dowdy, mother-of-the-bride look, those pastel suits with a lacy long-sleeved jacket and ankle-length matching skirt. Finally, I find something perfect. An above-the-knee, off-white sheath dress, made in a beautiful brocade fabric with a jewel neckline. I even find a satin headband to coordinate.

Resource: Consider a custom veil.

If you want a pretty head-cover on your wedding day, and prefer not to wear a wig or hat, check out chemobeanies.com. They can make a soft, beautiful white cloche with yards of netting and lace. Also, consider Anne Hathaway's lace-wrapped headpiece on her wedding day, a lovely solution to her shorn hair after she played Fantine in the film *Les Miserables*.

∼

It's challenging to feel attractive when your hair is a post-chemo, kinky mess. Or when you are missing a breast (or two), but I'm determined to try. I return to the Boobtique, where I select a pretty black satin nightgown with sewn-in pockets to accommodate the clone. Then I face the one task that can dishearten even the most enthusiastic shopper: choosing a swimsuit!

Normally, I'd try on dozens before finding anything. The selection here is actually much better than I expected. Still, I grit my teeth and face the mirror. The metallic silver tank makes me resemble a porpoise. The floral skirted suit makes me look like Great Aunt Ethel.

Not feeling optimistic, I'm happily surprised to find a cute turquoise tankini with matching sarong, cut low enough to escape being dowdy, yet high enough to conceal my scars and prosthesis. This will work just fine.

Leaving the Boobtique in an upbeat mood, I decide to color outside the lines and shop for something to "enhance the romance," like scented massage oil. However, I'm far too embarrassed to visit Adult Toy Superstore near the mall, where I might run into an acquaintance. Instead, I drive to Tacky Lingerie Shop, located in a decrepit shopping center. I check my wallet to make sure I have cash, terrified of ending up on some kinky mailing list if I use my credit card.

Behind the tinted windows of my minivan, I put on sunglasses and scope out the parking lot, making sure I don't recognize anyone. I try to slip in unnoticed, but a bell attached to the door jangles.

"Hi, there!" The older woman greeting me has the gravelly voice and nicotine scent of a chain smoker. Her hair's bright yellow, her face plastered with thick, Tammy Faye Bakker–style makeup. "Can I help you?"

"I'm just browsing."

I look around, rather puzzled. Some items seem silly, others downright dangerous. I have absolutely no idea how some of these things are used, but I'm not about to ask.

Seedy Saleslady sneaks up behind me. "Check this out! Isn't it hilarious?"

"Oh, my!" I jump back in alarm. She's wearing an ankle-length apron illustrated with a cartoonish male physique, complete with a protruding 3D rubber penis.

"I've got a female one, too. Wanna looky?"

"Uh, I'll pass."

As I wander around the aisles, unnerved by the bizarre inventory, the front door jingles. Hopeful that Seedy Saleslady will be busy with another customer, I browse the shelves in the back of the store, searching for tamer merchandise.

"Hello there, missy!" I turn around and see Fat Redneck Guy. He's wearing faded jeans, a Nascar t-shirt, a trucker hat, and a smirk. He wiggles his unruly eyebrows. "Whatcha looking for? Need advice?"

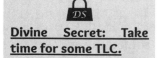

Divine Secret: Take time for some TLC.

Marriage is not for sissies! Cancer hasn't been a cakewalk for your partner, either. Take time to appreciate and rekindle your relationship.

"No, thank you," I answer, my Southern manners rising to the occasion. Aware that my etiquette might not be the only thing aloft, I back away from the leering stranger. I bump into a display of French-maid teddies, bob and weave around racks of bustiers and thong panties, dart past cases of neon-colored dildos and fuzzy handcuffs, then dash out the door.

I end up at Chain Drugstore. They have a smaller selection of massage oils, but there are no creepy dudes stalking me. I put two bottles in my shopping cart, under a giant bag of potato chips and some paper towels, in an effort to hide my naughty merchandise.

Resources: Spice up your wardrobe.

• Swimwear—For stylish, sexy swimwear designed to hide post-surgical scars and provide breast form pockets, check out veronicabrett.com and L.L.Bean at llbean.com.

• Nightgowns—Check out weaease.com and stillyou.com for pretty post-mastectomy nightgowns and pajamas.

• Nordie's—Nordstrom's lingerie department will add prosthetic breast pockets to their bras and nightgowns, offering more pretty choices.

• Camisoles—perfectcami.com has a large variety of lovely, light-weight camisoles that can extend your wardrobe options.

Twenty Years of Wedded... Er...Bliss

Ryan spent hours trying to redeem his frequent flier miles for airline tickets. He finally managed to score two free economy-class tickets to Europe. But since he had to schedule around black-out dates, we need to leave a few days earlier than we'd initially planned and fly into Paris rather than Venice, the cruise departure port. *So not a problem!*

We arrive in Paris jetlagged but excited. Thanks to Ryan's frequent guest program, we're booked into a very swanky hotel near the Opera House using his reward points. To save a few bucks, we avoid the taxi stand and catch an airport shuttle bus into the city, then schlep several blocks to the hotel. The lobby is gorgeous, with enormous crystal chandeliers and gilt-framed mirrors. I try to blend in with the limousine-chauffeured guests milling around the marble floors with their Prada and Chanel shopping bags. But our arrival, dragging suitcases down the sidewalk, tips everyone off that we are neither minor Scandinavian royalty nor international pop stars.

Over the next few days, we sip coffee at sidewalk cafés, visit Notre Dame, stroll the banks of the Seine, and admire the Eiffel Tower. Hard to find a more scenic, romantic setting than the City of Love—even if we decline pricey room-service breakfasts, buying our chocolate croissants from a chain bakery in the subway instead.

But on the third day, Ryan has reached his lovey-dovey limit. While touring the Louvre, he reverts to an obsessed photo-taking American tourist, missing only the white socks and black sandals. Caught up in a Kodak-induced frenzy, he walks ahead of me to snap yet another picture of yet another statue. Finally, my patience runs out.

"Slow down!" I plead. "This is our *anniversary* vacation. Not a photography field trip."

"You're right." Sheepish, he grabs my hand.

We spend our last night in Paris at a charming bistro near Montmartre, on a hill overlooking the city lights. Seated at a linen-clad table, we have a front-row seat for people watching. Crowds wander around the square, admiring artists as they daub paint on canvas.

"Guess what?" I say. "I have an anniversary surprise!"

"You do? But I didn't get you anything. I thought this trip was our gift."

"It is. The surprise is something different." I pause, my stomach fluttery with excitement. "I've made plans to renew our marriage vows on the ship!"

"Oh?" He looks puzzled. "I didn't think they'd expired."

"They didn't." I look down at my plate of sautéed chicken and pommes frites. "I thought it might be fun."

I can't help feeling deflated. Hidden in my garment bag is the ivory brocade sheath I'd purchased for the occasion.

"I'm sorry." Ryan reaches over and gives me a hug. "It *does* sound like fun."

I swallow the lump in my throat. "Things have been tough lately, so I thought…"

"It's a great idea!" he insists. "You caught me off guard, that's all." He leans across the table and kisses me.

After dinner, we sit on the steps of Sacré-Cœur, gazing at the lights of Paris. I savor the sweetness of the moment and try to ignore the challenges ahead. We haven't sailed out of

Cancerland yet. I face reconstruction, boatloads of doctor appointments, and years of taking anti-recurrence medication. But we've made it this far without cancer being an iceberg to our Titanic.

~

We fly to Venice and board our cruise, watching as the ship sails away from the crumbling yet magnificent city of canals. A few days later, we arrive at Mykonos, a picturesque Greek island. Today we plan to visit some Greek ruins in the morning and renew our vows in the late afternoon.

Before leaving for our tour, we have breakfast on the ship. On our way out, Ryan casts a longing glance at the buffet.

I can read his mind. "No, honey," I say. "We are not pilfering bananas, bagels, and little boxes of Captain Crunch for a picnic lunch. We are going to eat at one of those overpriced outdoor cafés like all the other tourists."

Since it is a special day, Ryan does not argue.

~

Late that afternoon, looking at a panoramic backdrop of domed white houses and a turquoise blue sea, we renew our wedding vows as the ship departs Mykonos. It's a private moment, with only the cruise ship official, events hostess, and photographer present.

Standing together, I think about the words we repeated twenty years ago.

For better or worse. For richer or poorer. In sickness and in health.

The first time we said those words, we were in our mid-20s, just a few years out of college, with hopes and dreams of a bright future together. Our relationship is solid, but like most married couples, we've had our disagreements, misunderstandings, and petty annoyances.

But throughout all our years together, there's always been love and trust.

As we navigate through the "in sickness and in health" part, I'll admit neither of us have been stellar role models for cancer survivorship. Many times I retreated to the bedroom or stayed glued to my computer, disengaged from our kids, caught up in my own emotions and anxieties. Ryan became extra control-freaky, obsessing over homework and trivial household matters, often losing sight of the big picture.

Despite the challenges, we're here today, together and happy.

The cruise official, a young lady in a navy blue suit and a gold name tag, begins the ceremony. I'd arranged the vow renewal as sort of a lark, a fun event to mark the occasion, but now strong emotions of relief and gratitude bubble to the surface. *I'm going to be around for many more anniversaries.*

"Today we are here to renew your vows of loyalty and love."

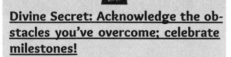

Divine Secret: Acknowledge the obstacles you've overcome; celebrate milestones!

Relationships are challenging. I know some Pink Sisters whose partners bailed, unwilling or unable to cope with the stress of cancer. In tough times, character shines through. If your partner turned out to be a selfish, shallow jerk during your treatment, he was probably a selfish, shallow jerk beforehand. You deserve better! But even in a good relationship, it's doubtful that your partner could fulfill all your emotional needs. He probably didn't always say the right thing or perform certain tasks exactly the way you wanted. But if your partner has stood beside you, even if imperfectly, celebrate your love.

Ryan and I look at each other. We've each gained a few pounds and some wrinkles since he waited by the altar as I walked down the aisle in my puffy satin wedding gown. Over the past twenty years, we've built a family and created memories.

"Ryan and Joanna, will you re-commit yourself to one another, renewing your vows of love and loyalty?"

Our words are spoken in unison. "We will."

"Will you promise to laugh with each other in

joy and grieve with each other in sorrow?"

Smiling, we repeat the pledge. Our eyes start to tear.

"Will you promise to hold hands as you walk together through life?"

Ryan and I pause for a millisecond, remembering the Louvre. We start to snicker, then burst out laughing. The cruise ship lady raises her eyebrows.

"Private joke," I explain.

"But we will," adds Ryan.

We're instructed to kiss, and after a sweet smooch, Ryan envelopes me in a hug. Rather than being cheesy, like a Vegas wedding chapel with an Elvis impersonator, the ceremony is a joyful, exhilarating moment. After toasting with champagne and chocolate-covered strawberries, we pose for photos at scenic locations throughout the ship. Later that evening, at the ship's private party for honeymooners and couples celebrating anniversaries, we're asked to cut the cake and take the floor for the symbolic first dance.

Divine Secret: Money can't buy you love.

Maybe you don't have enough time off or money to book a vacation. But celebrating your relationship doesn't have to be pricey. Consider a quiet picnic in a beautiful park. Plan a reenactment of your first date when you ate pizza and went skating. Work together on a project, such as compiling a photo DVD set to music of family memories.

What Happens In Vegas

We return home, and the kids are glad to see us, especially when they realize we've bought them souvenirs. Mom is even happier to see us, exhausted after babysitting our five children: three human, two canine.

I didn't know how prophetic my words to Foster Dog Mom would be; indeed, Rover fits in perfectly with the rest of our dysfunctional clan. Haunted by memories as a hungry stray, he eats whatever we put in front of him and has grown as round as a barrel. Insecure and neurotic, he's started marking his territory. To break him of this habit, I've been keeping him close at my side, even at times making him wear silly-looking "poochie pants"—little plaid overalls for doggies with incontinence issues.

Overcome with excitement at seeing his master and mistress, Rover sprays a dining chair leg. I immediately grab paper towels and cleaning supplies. Back to reality; vacation is over!

"Bad dog, Rover!" Mom fusses. "No, no!"

Rover appears chastened, his tail between his legs, floppy ears flattened, big brown eyes remorseful.

"He's not a bad dog!" I say. "He's a good dog who makes bad choices."

Karen, a friend and former colleague, calls. Though we've exchanged e-mails sporadically, it's been several years since we've spoken. After chatting for a few minutes, her voice deepens.

"Joanna, I have sad news. Carl's dead."

"Oh, no!" Our team had worked together on numerous projects, becoming friends as well as co-workers, laughing over lunches and happy hours.

"What happened?"

Karen hesitates. "He committed suicide. Put a gun to his head."

I feel like throwing up. *This makes no sense!*

Carl was a quiet but friendly guy, with some persnickety habits, sort of like Ryan. We'd been the office *Odd Couple*; he was the Felix to my Oscar.

"Why?"

"I heard marital issues. And financial problems."

This is hard to understand. Carl was well respected by his colleagues, and he had a daughter he adored. I hang up the phone, shaking my head. I've spent months in the oncologist's office, in hospitals, in infusion centers, surrounded by people fighting for their lives, hoping for more time.

I ache deep inside, heartbroken that no one could save Carl from his despair.

~

Larissa and I fly to Las Vegas for a reunion with our adoption travel group. It's been five years since we brought our daughters home from China, four years since our last reunion at Myrtle Beach. I wish Ryan and the boys could be here, too, but our vacation budget is bankrupt. Thank goodness we had enough remaining airline miles for two free tickets.

Vegas probably isn't the first place you'd think of for a kid-friendly gathering, yet it offers a variety of family-oriented activities. We steer clear of the casinos and topless showgirls, choosing to explore Red Rock Canyon, splash in the swimming pool, ride kiddie coasters at Circus Circus, and watch sharks at the Mandalay Bay aquarium. I'm especially glad that Christine's husband Jeff and their two daughters Emma and Isabelle have joined us. It's been a tough road for their family, but the girls are happy and thriving.

En route to yet another fun-filled outing, Jeff retrieves the rental car from the parking garage while Larissa and I stand in a shady spot with the girls.

"Hey, Emma," I say. "Love your outfit!"

"Thanks!" She gives me a big grin. "Everyone says I have a lot of style. Just like my Mommy."

"Why isn't your mommy here?" asks Larissa.

I cringe, sorry for the words that must pierce their hearts. I'd talked to Larissa beforehand, but apparently she's forgotten.

"Our mom died a few years ago. Back when we were little." Isabelle's calm reply reveals that she's used to answering this question.

"I knew your mommy and liked her very much," I say. "Everyone did. She was smart, beautiful, and kind. Just like you girls. She'd be so proud of you both."

They light up with smiles.

"And you're absolutely correct, Emma. Your mom had fabulous style. Obviously, you've inherited her flair!"

By the time Jeff returns, the girls are comparing their hair accessories. We get our daughters buckled in while they tune their headphones to the latest Carrie Underwood CD.

On the drive to our next event, Jeff and I talk.

"How are you doing?" he asks. "Health wise?"

"I'm fine now. Facing reconstructive surgery, then I'll be done."

"So it's early-stage? Good outlook?"

"That's what my doctors say."

"Glad to hear it."

"I hate cancer. It's so sneaky and random." I turn my head toward the backseat, where the girls are bobbing their heads to the beat. "I mean, look at Christine. She was a runner, a vegetarian, someone in top shape."

"Yeah, it was a total surprise. And we thought she had it beat."

"I know it's been tough. But you're an awesome dad. The girls are great."

"Yeah, they are," he says, glancing in the rearview mirror as the girls start singing the chorus, something about bashing headlights with a Louisville Slugger.

During the drive, we recount our unwelcome adventures in Cancerland. It feels good to talk about Christine.

"We miss her every day," he admits. "But a few good things have happened. The girls are super close to their grandparents. And their cousins."

"Got to search for those silver linings."

"I agree," he nods. "I'll take whatever silver linings I can find."

Despite carrying grief, they're moving forward. I'm sure that's what Christine would have wanted.

Divine Secret: Say their names.

People are often reluctant to bring up the name of someone who has died, worried about stirring up grief. But the feelings of bereavement are already there, so ignoring the loss causes a different kind of hurt. Talking about loved ones we miss may be painful, but it's also sweetly comforting.

♡52 Did I Pass or Fail?

My BRCA test results are back, so I meet with the geneticist, a friendly woman with a crisp and confident manner. At our previous appointment, she reviewed my personal and family medical histories and ordered my blood sample. Unlike with my stereotactic biopsy, this time I'm smart enough to receive the potentially bad news in person, rather than over the phone.

Confident Geneticist escorts me to a small conference room, where she introduces me to an oncologist and a social worker, both also female. She opens a manila folder and hands me a brochure from the testing lab.

"I've got your results. I can tell you that it's good news."

But her guarded expression concerns me.

"You did *not* test positive for any of the known BRCA1 or BRCA2 genes linked to breast or ovarian cancer. That's great news."

I look at the oncologist and social worker. Their smiles also seem restrained.

"Okay." I read over the paper she's handed me. Hmm, my outcome does not say "Negative."

"I'm confused. What does *Variant of Unknown Significance, Favors Polymorphism, Not Deleterious* mean?"

"You have a result that about ten percent of people receive. *Variant of Unknown Significance* means they found a mutation in your BRCA cells. The term *Favors Polymorphism* means the lab believes the variant is not harmful, but needs more data to confirm."

"So this put me in a gray area, right? Since the report is not clearly *Negative* or *Positive*?"

"Many high-risk families test negative for known BRCA1 and BRCA2 deleterious mutations. With your mother's diagnosis, you do have some family history. Even if someone has a negative BRCA test result, that doesn't mean there's not a genetic connection. There's much we don't know yet."

She explains that the scientific community has only scratched the surface of genetic testing, and that they are learning new things every day.

But why, oh why, do all of **my** *medical decisions have to be so difficult? I'm sick of ambivalent, confusing test results.*

"The lab is actively collecting data on your gene variant to learn more. They're offering to test your parents and siblings for free."

The BRCA test normally costs over $3,000. They must be seriously interested in pursuing further investigation. I read the explanation on my report once again. They've only seen this particular variant 17 times.

I'm no geneticist—Botany 101 in college was as far as I got—but they don't seem to have enough information on my variant to determine anything for certain.

"I don't know. I think I'm still leaning toward a prophylactic mastectomy."

The three women nod and don't say anything to discourage me. Confident Geneticist has been spouting the official party line, but I sense that they understand my uneasiness.

~

As soon as I get home, I call Mom.

"Hey, how are you feeling?" She's been going to the plastic surgeon every week or two to have her tissue expander filled with more saline water, preparing for the breast implant.

"Good! That first fill hurt like heck, but this one wasn't bad."

"Well, I got my BRCA results back."

"What did they say?"

"I tested negative for the known BRCA1 and BRCA2 gene mutations. But they did find a gene variant. They don't think it's harmful, but they can't confirm that."

"Really?"

"I'm so tired of feeling confused! Why can't anything be simple?"

"I know."

"My report said they'd only seen this variant seventeen times. The lab is offering to test you for free. I have some paperwork to give to your doctor."

"Okay. Put it in the mail."

"This is the tipping point. I definitely want the prophylactic mastectomy. I don't want to spend the rest of my life worrying."

"I don't blame you."

Divine Secret: Sometimes a medical test will NOT give you a clear answer.

Sometimes test results only add to your confusion and frustration. All you can do is keep asking questions until you're sure you've reached your best decision.

Smart Doctors and Not-So-Smart Friends

Fall 2008

The kids start another school year. Determined to get my mojo back, I agree to volunteer in my neighbor's third-grade classroom and to help out with Girl Scouts. With Alex on the track team, Nick playing basketball, and Larissa signed up for soccer, we all stay busy with sporting events and practices.

Since so much of my time revolves around kid activities, it's a treat to hang out with grown-ups from time to time. I find myself at a small party, in the kitchen sampling the desserts, when the hostess starts to rave about how much she loves her recent cosmetic breast reduction and lift.

"One of the best experiences in my life!" she crows. "Right up there with my wedding and the births of my children."

I stand there, lopsided and scarred, a silicone triangle shoved into one side of my bra. Unable to think of an appropriate reply, I pop another cheesecake bite into my mouth.

She knows what I've been going through. *Did she forget? Maybe she thinks I'll be inspired by her success story, even though reconstruction and reduction procedures have nothing in common.*

However, since she's not a mean-spirited person, I give her a Stupid Pass.

Sometimes smart individuals can say really dumb things, so I keep those metaphorical Stupid Passes handy. I can't believe how many people reel off a litany of relatives, colleagues, and acquaintances who've succumbed to cancer. *Way to cheer a girl up, folks!*

Perhaps it's their misguided attempt at empathy, to somehow connect. At the very least, the lists people share of their dearly departed remind me that, someday, all of us will face heartbreak and loss.

∼

At my next appointment with Rock Star Surgeon, I tell him that, after factoring in my mom's diagnosis and my fuzzy BRCA results, I definitely want a prophylactic mastectomy. He no longer tries to dissuade me; I've had plenty of time to think it over. I also tell him I don't want to use wishy-washy Dr. Quizzical. Caring Nurse assures me she'll schedule an appointment with a different plastic surgeon.

I don't bring up my feelings, also factored into my decision, though intangible. They cannot be calculated on a spreadsheet, only seen through a personal rubric. Some women who test positive for BRCA1 or BRCA2 genes, with a sizeable known risk of cancer, call themselves "pre-vivors" and choose to have their breasts or ovaries removed proactively. Others decide to hope for the best or postpone surgery, opting for frequent surveillance and screening.

At times, I may differ in opinion with my Pink Sisters, but I will always respect their choices. Also, though this may seem shallow to some, having good symmetry is important to me. I want a matched set! The discrepancy between a perky "foob" on the right and a naturally-aging breast on the left seems depressing, a constant reminder of the cancer. As the years go by, the difference becomes even more pronounced. At some point, the clothing label name "Sag Harbor" would be quite apropos.

∼

Ryan accompanies me to my appointment with Dr. L'Artiste, a plastic surgeon with a thick French-Canadian accent. As usual, I've google-stalked Dr. L'Artiste, pleased to learn he specializes in reconstructive surgeries, treating not only cancer survivors, but people born with facial deformities or who've been injured in car accidents.

With simple blue-gray chairs and a TV bolted to the wall, his office looks more like a typical medical facility, less like a country club, which immediately makes me more comfortable.

Dr. L'Artiste steps into the exam room and introduces himself. He's a handsome man with a pleasant but serious vibe. After a brief exam, he explains how he would surgically implant two saline-filled expanders under my chest muscles. Every other week, more saline water would be added, gradually stretching out the skin and muscle enough to make a pocket for the breast implant. At that point, he'd surgically swap out the expanders for implants. Dr. L'Artiste goes on to explain that many women require an additional small procedure or two, to add nipples or make minor revisions.

"Would you like to see zee photos?"

"Yes, please." We'll get to see his work! I grin at Ryan.

Dr. L'Artiste hands me a thick album.

"Merci beaucoup!" I say, lapsing into my college French 101.

He raises a Gallic eyebrow. I wonder if Rock Star Surgeon's office has warned him I'm a bit nutty.

I flip through the pages. I've read that women who undergo delayed reconstruction are often happier with their results than those who get immediate reconstruction. I wonder why this is. Would you wake up dismayed by the appearance and feeling of the expanders? Maybe, mourning the loss of your natural breasts, you'd be disappointed. But after months or years spent dealing with prosthetic breasts, pocketed bras, blouses with higher armholes or necklines, maybe women undergoing delayed reconstruction are pleased to have "foobs," even if less than perfect.

Browsing through Dr. L'Artiste's photos, I decide his results are quite satisfactory. I'd be happy with a similar outcome.

"Those look nice." Ryan points to a photo.

"You realize we're not ordering from a catalog?"

He gives me an innocent expression. "Just offering my opinion."

At one point, I'd had my heart set on a DIEP procedure—and the bonus tummy tuck—but I'm impressed by how good Dr. L'Artiste's patient photos look.

I tug at the album, but Ryan has it firmly in his grasp.

"Let go, please!" I roll my eyes.

I ask Dr. L'Artiste a number of questions: *Were these implants saline or silicone? High-profile or moderate profile? What cup size are the breasts in this picture?*

The surgeon answers my questions, explaining that profile refers to the depth or projection of the implants and that, since so much tissue is removed, most reconstruction patients need the high profile. He hands us samples made with saline versus silicone for show-and-tell. Both the orbs are liquid-filled, but the silicone version seems squishier. I know Mom is choosing a saline implant, but I'm leaning toward silicone, more commonly used in breast reconstruction.

Divine Secret: Surgeons may use different "Build-a-Boob" techniques.

Not every good doctor is going to have the exact same approach. Mom's surgeon—whom she loved—wrapped her post-surgical torso with ACE-type bandages like a mummy, whereas Rock Star Surgeon affixed a piece of surgical tape over my scar. Mom went with saline implants; I chose silicone. Differences in the details, but we're both happy with our results.

Before we finish, I pose for yet another topless photo. Pleased with what we've seen and heard, I tell Dr. L'Artiste I'd like to schedule a surgery date for a prophylactic mastectomy and bilateral reconstruction.

Update: Silicone gel implants are a new option.

Some of my Pink Sisters have nicknamed these the "Gummy Bear" option. Ask your plastic surgeon for advice. Compared to the liquid silicone implants, the gelatin-filled implants may offer a more natural feel and reduced chance of leakage in case of rupture.

Resources:

For more information about implants, check out these manufacturer websites:

* allergan.com
* mentorwwllbc.com

Survivor Sibling Rivalry

At my next follow-up with Dr. Point Guard, I complain about the increased number of migraines triggered by the aromatase inhibitor he prescribed. Although it's not an issue in my case, I know a lot of women struggle with joint and bone pain on AIs. For some the side effects were so severe that they stopped taking the drug; others managed to muddle through. Because my headaches can be excruciating, Dr. Point Guard recommends that I switch back to tamoxifen, a drug I tolerated quite well.

No one wants a recurrence, but I'm suddenly aware that every survivor has to draw her personal line in the sand. What will she do? What will she not do? What drugs/treatments can she tolerate? Which ones are problematic? What healthy lifestyle changes is she willing to make?

I ask Dr. Point Guard whether he plans to schedule me for a PET scan, a highly-sensitive test to pick up suspected abnormalities anywhere within your body. Some of my Pink Sisters have this done on a regular basis.

"No, I don't order routine scans," Dr. Point Guard says, shaking his head. "Not for someone in your situation, with early-stage cancer. It's used more for metastatic disease to evaluate treatment and measure progression."

"You don't?" *After all this time and effort spent trying to eradicate cancer cells, all I get is blood work and a physical?*

"Studies have shown that finding tumors from routine PET scans, rather than after symptoms are present, does not lead to any significant difference in outcome, meaning length of survival."

"That doesn't make sense." I'm baffled by the differing policies for follow-up. Rock Star Surgeon told me I won't need mammograms anymore since most of my breast tissue is gone; Mom's doctor is still scheduling them for her. Maybe some oncologists perform routine scans, others don't.

"I know it's hard to grasp, but survival rates stay the same after symptoms present, whether or not the tumor was spotted through a routine PET scan while asymptomatic or while investigating after a problem shows up. Basically, that means knowing about the tumor will not give you any more time. You'd discover the Stage IV cancer earlier, but wouldn't necessarily live any longer. Also, PET scans are very sensitive, but not very specific. Which means a lot of false positives."

"So, my follow-up is basically blood work and a physical exam? That's it?"

"Yes, but if you ever show troubling symptoms, I'll order a scan right away. Keep in mind the two-week rule. If you have any concerning indicator—unexplained pain, persistent fever, etc.—that doesn't resolve in two weeks, you should give me a call."

Okay, that sounds reasonable. Call Dr. Point Guard when I have a problem that doesn't get better in two weeks. Scan when there is a suspicious symptom, not on a routine screening basis. With my neurotic

Divine Secret: Scan-xiety is normal.

Although not recommended for me, some Pink Sisters will undergo regularly scheduled scans. They've dubbed the accompanying fear and stress as "scan-xiety." Expect your nerves to be rattled, and figure out a plan to cope, whether through meditation, relaxation tapes, talks with other survivors, even an occasional Ativan.

imagination, I'd probably face enormous "scan-xiety" over every test, worrying myself sick over every minor anomaly. I want to live my life looking forward, not over my shoulder with fear and trepidation.

~

Some Pink Sisters develop close friendships with local survivors, but with Ryan's business travel and the kids' sporting events, it's hard to make the weeknight meetings. Instead, I share my deepest, scariest thoughts with my *YSC* friends in cyberspace. Our online connections are powerful, and I'm glad I can seek out companionship any time, day or night. Also, my virtual friends understand when I get overwhelmed and have to take a mental break for a day, a week, or a month.

Though many women become close pals through the process, I'm wary of befriending a Pink Sister living close enough to meet for lunch or shopping. *Would our strongest common bond always be cancer? Would that person be a constant reminder of the hard times?*

Not that I'm such a prize BFF. I can be a mediocre friend. If I haven't married you, given birth to you, or adopted you, I probably won't remember your birthday. Not one for frequent phone chats, I'll let time slip away between conversations. My most intimate friends tend to be low maintenance, with powerful senses of humor and streaks of wackiness. But they've been there for me. Mary Lou called and e-mailed often, sent pajamas, slippers, tiny pillows, and books. Although her dad's a Presbyterian minister, Beth sent a prayer shawl blessed by a Catholic priest, because it never hurts to have a back-up plan!

On the plus side, if you're nice to my family, you're in my friendship circle. Life changes and people move away. But if you were my friend in high school, college, or our young married days, I still hold you close in my heart.

Despite my flaws, I've never battled the "green-eyed monster."

Whenever something good happens to a friend—swanky vacation, fabulous promotion, gorgeous new house—I'm sincerely happy for her, never jealous.

That is, until Sunny Survivor.

I would include Sunny Survivor in my wide circle of friends. She's a bright, attractive, vivacious person sparkling with energy and enthusiasm. After my first surgery, she brought over a delicious chicken casserole and homemade apple pie.

When I hear she's been diagnosed with cancer (not breast), I feel terrible. *I hate fricking cancer!* Over the next two weeks, every single day I have good intentions to call her. Yet I stare at the phone, my fingers paralyzed. I can't do it.

Suddenly, I understand Teal Ribbon Mom's radio silence. She'd sounded so eager to help me, but then she never returned my calls. Now I get it. Deep inside, cancer leaves a visceral fear behind, threatening to pop up like a demented jack-in-the-box. I don't want to think about cancer or talk about it. Never brave, I was just bluffing, using humor as a shield.

When Sunny Survivor calls, wanting to ask some chemotherapy questions, I feel lower than dirt. I should have forced myself to pick up the phone first. A day later, guilty with remorse, I drop off brownies, along with hats and scarves I no longer need.

I send cards and e-mails as she goes through treatment. We meet for coffee a few times, comparing our experiences. I share my Stupid Pass philosophy. She jokes about the dubious fringe benefits of having cancer.

"Whenever I go to lunch with friends, they always say something to the waiter. And I get a free dessert."

"Awesome." I nod in agreement. "Nothing wrong with playing the Cancer Card. I'd do it for a slice of key lime pie or turtle cheesecake."

Though, to be honest, I've been playing the Cancer Card plenty. After her first chemo, Sunny Survivor volunteered to serve snacks at the middle school dance. After my first treatment, I stayed home in my pajamas, reading a book about teenaged vampires.

Divine Secret: Survivorship is not a competition.

We each have our own path to follow through Cancerland. Nobody's perfect; don't compare your accomplishments to those of others. Realize you might be coping with some post-traumatic stress and give yourself time. Many Pink Sisters eventually volunteer to help those newly diagnosed, but at first, revisiting thoughts of the disease can be too painful. Give yourself a break.

I can't help these strange, unsettling feelings, even though I like her. My insides burn when I think about her well-adjusted family. Her husband has a calm, unflappable demeanor, unlike Ryan, who gets stressed and control-freaky. Sunny Survivor's kids are model students, unfailingly polite. When the principal calls, it's because one of them has won a spelling bee or citizenship award. But when a principal calls me, it's usually a behavior issue, like the time Nick—using the classroom computerized dictionary, which pronounces and defines words—cranked up the volume and typed in p–e–n–i–s, horrifying his prim and proper teacher. I hate feeling jealous; it's an ugly sensation. And to be jealous of a fellow cancer survivor, that's pathetic!

A Strange Soliloquy

At 16 months past my cancer diagnosis, I'm scheduled for reconstructive surgery in a few weeks. But until then, I'm squeezing in as many fun, active days as possible.

For my second Komen race, I organize a team of about a dozen members. This time, several friends, as well as Nick and Alex, want to run competitively, so they attach timer chips to their shoelaces. The rest of us decide to walk.

The downtown streets are packed with participants, buzzing with an excited, caffeinated vibe. Sponsors hand out bagels, bananas, and water bottles. Worried about regrouping after the race, I wear a pink sequin cowgirl hat. This works better than expected. The sun bounces off the tiny reflective discs, blinding bystanders. *No one can miss me now!* I hand out pink feather boas to my team members. Getting in the spirit, Nick dons Larissa's pink rhinestone-accented sunglasses.

The serious runners stretch their legs and weave through the crowd, edging closer to the starting line, while the slowpokes stay further back. When the whistle blows, the race starts with a positive, high-energy pace. Young and old, male and female, fit and flabby all crowd the streets. Parents push strollers festooned with pink streamers. Some teams wear matching tie-dyed t-shirts or floppy hats. A group of guys run in dresses, accessorized with costume jewelry and handbags, eliciting giggles and applause.

Yet, underneath the laughter and high spirits is a sad underpinning, the bittersweet acknowledgement of those lost. My eyes are drawn to the signs safety-pinned to many backs: "Running in Memory of ____," the names scrawled in black marker. I think of my beautiful departed *YSC* sisters—e.g. Lola, DKNY, Danica—who offered support and encouragement while enduring their Stage IV battles. I never hugged them in person, but our hearts embraced through the long stretches of the information highway.

After crossing the finish line, I walk toward the stage area, where I'm joined by the rest of my team members. Since I'm wearing the official pink survivor shirt, I receive a special swag bag filled with goodies—one of the few perks of being in the sisterhood. We walk around, sampling Skinny Cow ice cream bars and other freebies.

Volunteers armed with pink helium balloons work their way through the crowd, preparing for the closing ceremony. I get a balloon to mark the passage of time since my diagnosis. I look around, encouraged to see some women holding a dozen or more, all bobbing in the cool breeze.

After an announcement of how much money was raised by today's race, someone reads a poem over the loudspeaker. Survivors release their helium balloons, lifting up unspoken hopes and prayers, turning the sky into a beautiful pink mosaic.

~

As Ryan and I drive to the hospital in the pre-dawn darkness, the atmosphere is very different from the last time. My mood is upbeat, free of the grim fear that hovered over me before previous surgeries. Today, Rock Star Surgeon will perform a prophylactic mastectomy, and then Dr. L'Artiste will insert two tissue expanders under my chest muscles. With drains on both sides,

I won't be able to drive or lift anything for a while.

I wake up in the recovery area with Ryan standing next to me. Underneath the bandages on my chest, I can see two small bumps. After a few hours, I'm wheeled to my room. A pleasant nurse introduces herself, gives me the "Service Excellence" spiel, and asks me who performed my surgery.

Still groggy, I mumble their names.

"Wow, you've got the Dream Team!"

Smiling, I drift off to sleep.

~

My hospital stay lasts a few days. The friendly staff introductions, mindless TV shows, and trays of mystery meat with green jello are now routine. But once I go home, disconnected from the pain pump, I feel like someone's shoved a pair of Tupperware sandwich containers into my chest. My right underarm area, where sentinel nodes were removed, aches constantly. With the surgical drains, I can't wear a bra comfortably. (Not that I'd need one, since I'm now an AA cup size.) I've signed on for months of discomfort to have a semblance of what Fergie from The Black Eyed Peas calls "those lovely lady lumps."

Throughout history, women have suffered in pursuit of beauty. I think of the little girls in ancient China with bound, broken feet. Teenaged Zulu girls with their necks stretched out like giraffes by stacks of metal rings. Even today, plenty of women tolerate scratchy contact lenses and pinchy stilettos. I'm drawn to the mirror, so happy to no longer see a lopsided reflection. Naturally busty before cancer, I often felt self-conscious. It's liberating not to have so much weight on my chest.

~

After a week of recovery, still sore and medicated, hiding drains under a baggy blouse, I bum a ride to the first-grade field trip with neighbors. Larissa wants me to go to the Gem Mine, and

I don't want to disappoint her. The two moms in the car, both cheerful blondes, are very nice, but I don't know them well.

"How are you feeling these days?" asks Carpool Mom #1.

"Okay, but not great. I can't drive yet, so I appreciate the lift."

"Anytime."

"My mom battled breast cancer," confides Carpool Mom #2. "She had reconstruction, too. So, are you done with your surgeries?"

"Not yet. I'll have one when I get the implants. After that, maybe another."

Still loopy from my prescriptions, I launch into a lengthy "to nip or not to nip" soliloquy, pondering aloud the pros and cons as well as the various techniques of nipple reconstruction and tattooing.

Uh-oh. I've been rambling on for quite some time.

The two women are completely silent.

Awkward!

"I'm so sorry! Just did some major over-sharing!"

"That's okay," Carpool Mom #1 says. "It's interesting."

"No need to apologize, nothing wrong with talking about it," adds Carpool Mom #2.

I appreciate that they're trying to make me feel better, but I still feel like an idiot. Nipples are a completely appropriate conversation topic among Pink Sisters, but not so much with girls who haven't pledged the sorority.

~

A week later, I've stopped taking prescription pain meds, so I resume driving, but have to take Alex or Nick with me to the grocery store to put heavy stuff—the milk cartons and boxes of canned soda—into the grocery cart. Walking around the supermarket is a big-time outing for me, since I have to limit activity to lessen fluid output and allow removal of the drains. Sitting around the house, it doesn't take long before I start to feel restless.

Despite the boredom, my mood is positive, and I look forward to completing the reconstruction process.

~

The weekend before Halloween, I volunteer at our neighborhood carnival, where I'm stationed behind the dessert table with Jogging Neighbor, who's also a Pink Sister.

After handing a chocolate chip cookie to a miniature superhero, she leans in next to me and whispers, "What are you going to do about nipples?"

A gypsy and a fairy step up to the dessert table before I can answer.

"Could I have a brownie?"

"Me too, please."

"Of course," I answer, handing them their treats.

"I don't know," I reply in hushed, furtive tones as they walk away.

A ghost, two witches, and a vampire approach.

"Rice Krispy treat, please."

"I'd like a cupcake."

"Here you go, sweetie," says Jogging Neighbor, as we fill their requests.

"Wow, you guys look scary!" I add.

When the coast is clear, we pick up our conversation.

"I'm not telling anyone what I'm doing." Jogging Neighbor has a defiant twinkle in her eye. "I'm so tired of other people thinking about my breasts! They're not public property!"

I nod in agreement. She's on to something. I decide to keep my nipple happenings undercover, too. Maybe I'll do nothing and live with smooth, Barbie-style foobs. Or have the "twist and stitch" technique performed. Or use donor tissue from my eyelid or groin area (ouch!).

I could follow the lead of some of my more free-spirited Pink Sisters and get whimsical tattoo designs instead. *Maybe Celtic knots? Or happy faces? Or daisies? Who knows? I might even copy rapper Kanye West, who replaced his bottom teeth with diamonds.* Now that would be some bling!

~

On Halloween night, Larissa balks at wearing the costume she picked out months ago.

"But honey, I thought you wanted to be Ariel."

"Not anymore."

"Why not?"

"I don't like those!" she cries, pointing to the mermaid's clam shell bra. "They scare me!"

My heart hurts. Larissa never seemed upset by my hair loss. In fact, she'd peek under my scarf and giggle. But it seems the idea of having breasts makes her fearful. Her body will start changing in just a few short years, and I don't want her to regard it as the enemy. *Damn cancer!*

"Mommy's okay," I say, embracing her in a hug. "You don't have to wear it if you don't want to. You've got plenty of other dress-up costumes." I can't help but wonder what emotions my daughter will struggle with as she grows and develops. And I think about my sons, too, worried about how this turbulent time in our lives has affected them.

Larissa changes into a light blue Cinderella gown and grabs her plastic pumpkin. Ryan accompanies her down the sidewalk, carrying a flashlight, while I head outside with my bowl of candy.

Neighbors have already set up their chairs in the cul-de-sac. I find a spot next to Sarah. We sample each other's candy and chat about our kids.

"May I ask you a really personal question? It might sound strange."

"Um, okay." She looks a bit uncertain. "Sure. Ask away."

"What's your bra size?"

A puzzled expression crosses her face. Then, she laughs. "34C."

"I thought so."

We stop talking, silenced by preschoolers holding out treat bags.

"Sorry," I say, during the next lull. "It was a really personal question. But I need to know what to aim for in my reconstruction. You're the perfect size, not too big, not too small."

"Why, thank you!" She raises her plastic cup of wine. "To your future boobs! May they turn out great!"

"Cheers," I say, lifting my own beverage.

"I never realized all that was involved in breast reconstruction."

"Yeah, and it's not cheap. By the time everything's done, my medical expenses for cancer treatment plus reconstruction may reach a hundred thousand dollars. Thank goodness insurance pays most of the bills."

"I'll say. When you're done, let's go shopping. No more cheapo discount bras for you!"

"Maybe I can get the Victoria's Secret diamond-studded pushup."

Sarah laughs. "You deserve it."

Divine Secret: You have the right to reconstruction.

Even if it's been decades since your mastectomy, the Women's Health and Cancer Rights Act (WHCRA), implemented in 1998, requires insurance companies, group health plans, and HMOs that cover mastectomy to also pay for reconstructive breast surgery. Find more information at cancer.org, the website of the American Cancer Society.

Small, Medium, or Large?

Ryan and I are at Dr. L'Artiste's office, waiting for my first "fill." It's great to be symmetrical again and ditch the clone. My swelling has gone down, but the plastic expanders have an odd shape. Rather than Spongebob Squarepants, I look like Spongebob Squareboobs.

Dr. L'Artiste walks in with a huge syringe sporting a four-inch needle, scaled for a Brontosaurus rather than a mere mortal.

"Oh, my goodness!" I exclaim.

"Wow. That's really big," Ryan adds, the color draining from his face. *I hope he doesn't pass out!*

To my relief, the procedure is painless—albeit surreal—as the doctor injects saline water via a metal port. I watch my "foobs" increase in size, the process reminding me of the Crissy doll I received on Christmas in 1972. I would press her bellybutton and watch her hair grow from the top of her head.

A few Pink Sisters warned that the fills can really hurt, but only the first causes me significant discomfort. I'm starting to realize that people with troublesome side effects—whether from a procedure or medication—are more likely to post messages about their experience than someone who finds it a non-issue.

After several appointments, my "foobs" are visibly larger. Yet I'm confused by my appearance, not sure what to think. It's like looking into a distorted carnival mirror, impossible to see my reflection accurately.

Should I go bigger? Or smaller? Or is this size just right?

Ryan suggests super-sizing to extra-large, but I nix that idea. I start quizzing the nurses in Dr. L'Artiste's office, asking their opinions.

∿

After months of dowdy shirts, it's fun having more wardrobe choices. For Hannah and Will's casual Hanukkah/Christmas party, I wear nice jeans and a black velveteen blouse with a tastefully narrow but deep plunge.

I greet Hannah with a hug. "Watch out for my expanders. They could put out your eye."

She laughs. "Really?" Spurred on by a little liquid courage, she takes her index finger and gives my foobs a poke. "Wow! Those are rock hard."

Next thing I know, Liz and Winona join in. They're intrigued. Other party guests stare in shock at our foob-poking experiment, although it's definitely more clinical than kinky.

"Joanna said one of them could put out my eye, and I believe her," says Liz.

"Gives new meaning to the term over-the-shoulder-boulder-holder," adds Winona.

"Each one has a metal port for the fills. I could do some interesting party tricks with a magnet."

"I've got some upstairs," Hannah replies.

"No, I was joking! Joking!" I shake my head. "Not enough daiquiris in your blender for that. I'm not ready to be one of Letterman's Stupid Human Tricks."

∿

I decide to take a poll at my next book club meeting. After another fill, I'm still uncertain about my ideal foob size.

"What's your opinion of the girls? Should I stop now or go a little bigger?"

Sue chokes on her wine. "That's a question I wasn't expecting!"

Everyone laughs.

"C'mon, I need your advice."

"I think you're a terrific size," responds Sharon.

"You look good," adds Julie. "They're a nice fit for your frame."

"Or you could go a little bigger!" Rebecca suggests.

"Cancer's lousy," I admit, taking a bite of spinach dip. "But hey, at least I get a nice, new, perky rack as my consolation prize."

If someone else made this comment to me, it would sound obnoxious. But since I'm in the Pink Sorority, it's okay to laugh. Like how it's okay to make Aggie jokes if you're an Aggie. Or blonde jokes if you're a blonde. Unwritten rule: You have to be in the club.

We refill our wine glasses and segue into a discussion about which cosmetic surgeries we'd choose if we won the lottery.

Days later, on our way to another party, Ryan worries I've turned into the female version of Frank Luntz: the Gallup pollster of boob size.

"Honey, please stop asking everyone's opinion of your boobs. It's embarrassing."

Funny how a year ago, I was too self-conscious to type the word "breast" on my *CaringBridge* page. Now I can't stop conducting cup-size focus groups.

Right before Valentine's Day, I have a surgery date to swap to the squishy implants. At my pre-op appointment, I point out to Dr. L'Artiste how one expander has migrated closer to my armpit.

"I am Bob zee Builder, I can fix it!"

"He has triplet preschoolers," his nurse explains.

~

The swap surgery goes fine, but my upper chest is swollen, with no hint of cleavage. It's a quick recovery with minimal pain. I'm glad to have the implants done, but need patience for the next six weeks. I've been warned I won't know the results until all the swelling goes down.

At my first post-surgical appointment, Dr. L'Artiste gives me a thick owner's manual—sort of like the car version you keep in your glove compartment—with an ID card and serial number for each implant. *I feel like the bionic woman!*

When he gets the camera out to take photos, I realize I've gotten disturbingly comfortable posing for topless pictures. For a brief moment, I consider joking around: arching my back, pursing my lips, and fluffing my hair like a Playboy model. He'd probably add the word "delusional" to my electronic records.

~

Several weeks later we head to church. I finally have foobs and my hair has grown out, albeit in a rather unattractive mullet-like fashion. Life feels better and I am grateful. I remember one of my favorite Winston Churchill quotes: "If you are going through hell, keep going." I've been stranded in Cancerland for quite some time, but now I'm nearing the border, finding my way out.

After the service, I stand on the lawn, talking with Barry. "Great sermon today."

"Thanks. We haven't talked in a while. How are you doing?"

"I just had my last major surgery. Reconstruction is pretty much done!"

There's an awkward pause. Barry stares at the grass. Just like with Ryan, I can read Barry's mind. For a brief moment, he's tongue-tied, confused about the appropriate response. Would I welcome a compliment? Or be offended? He's not sure.

Laughing at his perplexed expression, I change the subject. "Since I'm done with hospitals for a while, you guys can take me off the prayer list." Every Sunday, a section of the church bulletin is reserved for the names of parishioners experiencing health or personal difficulties.

"Wish I would have known that earlier," he jokes. "You've been taking up too much space. We had to reduce the font this week to squeeze in all the names."

Divine Secret: Shrug off the self-consciousness.

We all have the same basic body parts; no need to feel embarrassed about yours. In order to keep the process more discreet, some women buy a padded bra in the size they expect to be and use post-surgical cutlet-style fillers while expanding. But I decided that it is what it is. By that point, I didn't really care whether or not someone noticed my variable boob size.

Renewal:

We Are Family...I've Got All My Sisters With Me

Medical Merry-Go-Round

Spring 2009

Stop, please! I'm ready to get off this medical merry-go-round.

Like all Pink Sisters, I worry about recurrence. Whenever I have a strange ache in my midsection, I fret, before remembering the previous day's pilates class.

The *good* thing about being a cancer survivor is that medical personnel take your complaints very seriously.

The *bad* thing about being a cancer survivor is that medical personnel take your complaints very seriously.

Pink Sister status may snag you a VIP ticket, like a *Disney Fastpass,* for prompt attention and testing. Of course, this might mean you get a ride inside a CT scanner, much scarier than Space Mountain.

Or maybe not.

∼

One morning, feeling icky from a sinus infection, I make an appointment to see the nurse practitioner at Dr. Earnest's office, my new PCP. While in the shower, I notice a blotchy red and purple spot on my right forearm, the cancer side. After getting dressed, I google a description of the mark.

The dark splotch on my arm has ragged borders and multiple colors, both red flags! *Could this be skin cancer? Or even metastatic breast cancer spread to my arm?*

When the nurse practitioner walks in the exam room, fear hovers over me like a flock of hungry vultures. "I'm a cancer survivor, so I'm really worried about this," I say, thrusting out my forearm.

"Hmm." She looks at it, a slight frown on her face. "Doesn't look like skin cancer or skin mets to me. It's more like a pinch mark."

"Oh." My face turns red as I remember a recent entanglement with a sweater zipper.

Moments later, I hear the nurse practitioner laughing in the hall. Surely she's added "crazy hypochondriac" to my electronic file.

~

I go for an appointment with Hip Neurologist, the doctor I've seen about my headaches for over a dozen years. When we first met, he wore his hair in a ponytail, and silky shirts more suited for a nightclub than an exam room. We've developed a friendly relationship, always spending a few minutes chatting about vacations, events in the news, our kids' schools, etc.

Today we talk about Dr. Point Guard.

"He's treating my cousin," says Hip Neurologist. "And I think he's one of the smartest people at this hospital."

"I agree. So how is treatment going?"

"Not great. Advanced stage," he replies. "But my cousin's a cool guy, a professional musician. He's been teaching me to play guitar."

"I'm sorry. But glad you're spending time together."

On his way out of the exam room, Hip Neurologist pauses at the door. "Take care, dude."

Dude? He called me "dude?"

Is my lack of estrogen obvious? Have I sprouted more mustache hairs? Or grown an Adam's apple? Then I realize the doctor used the term affectionately, for a long-established patient, knowing better than to use a politically incorrect endearment.

So many families wrestle with cancer. On the drive home, I think about Hip Neurologist's cousin, this man I've never met, spending his last weeks and months sharing his love of music with family and friends.

~

I sit at my computer, reflecting on the times in my journey when I felt confused, frustrated, or scared. I've heard that "giving back" is an essential component to healing. Nobody wants my burnt lasagna, but maybe sharing my story could help someone. Not because I have such brilliant insights, but to offer hope that if I, neurotic and flawed, stumbled through Cancerland, maybe you can, too.

But writing and reliving the past is a challenge. *Will I come across as an over-sharing idiot?* I don't want to be lumped in with Jennifer Love Hewitt, the actress who blabbed about gluing rhinestones to her va-jay-jay for some sexy bling. Granted, my story is very personal; it feels a little weird to share so much. Yet, I'm not embarrassed, because many Pink Sisters struggle with the same experiences and emotions. I want to reassure them they are not alone.

Some days I procrastinate, indulging in crazy daydreams: I'm the featured author for Oprah's book club! First, she flies me to Chicago for an appearance on her show. This requires shopping for an awesome, TV-worthy outfit. I can't spring for a pair of pricey Louboutins, but maybe cute pumps from Payless and a can of red spray paint will do the trick. Oprah and I hit it off, so she invites me to join her and Gayle for a girlfriends weekend at her Hawaiian estate. Next thing I know, Nate Berkus is remodeling my house.

But other times, I'm productive. Slowly, the scribbled yellow notepad turns into a stack of typed pages. Some days, jotting down the words is easy; other days, it's not. Sometimes reliving the past is too painful. I have to walk away from the keyboard, needing more time and distance.

~

After a lengthy struggle with his health, Beth's father passes away. I take a flight to Texas, arriving in time to accompany Beth to the funeral home where she picks up the urn with his ashes. Bill was a minister for many years, so the funeral home staff knew him well. They offer their deepest condolences, talking about what a good man he was.

That night, in a house filled with their extended relatives, I sit at a table with Beth's daughter, nephew, and brother, selecting pictures of Bill for a folding photo display. We smile at the black and white wedding portraits, the Kodak snapshots of Beth and her brothers as children on Christmas morning, the recent pictures taken with grandchildren. There are more photos than we can display, a visual timeline of a life well spent.

The next day, the church is packed with mourners. When Beth takes the podium, she talks about family traditions they shared, her dad reading the comics aloud, taking them out for a steak lunch after he'd concluded his Sunday morning duties. Her brother recounts a story of how their father, a man with a calm and patient temperament, once pummeled a refrigerator. He'd been pastoring a small Southern church at a time when racism flared. Several men in the congregation treated the African-American groundskeeper rudely, calling him by his first name or "Boy." Bill had insisted the congregation address him as "Mr. Jenkins" and show him the same respect they'd give each other. A few men refused to comply. Alone, Bill took out his anger on a Frigidaire.

There is sadness and grief in the church but also love and admiration for Bill and the memories he's left behind. I'm swimming in the shallow end of the theological pool, but I believe

Divine Secret: Don't imagine a zebra stampede!

An old medical school adage instructs interns, "When you hear hoofbeats, think horses, not zebras." Some cancer survivors, like me, obsess over every random symptom, the fear of recurrence haunting us. Try to take a deep breath and remind yourself that sometimes a fever, ache, or bruise is just a simple fever, ache, or bruise.

the gospel of Patrick Swayze in *Ghost* when his character says, "It's amazing, Molly. The love inside, you take it with you."

Bill—being an ordained Presbyterian minister—would have added the words of the apostle Paul that love "bears all things, believes all things, hopes all things, endures all things."

That sounds good, too.

Resource: Book

Living Well Beyond Breast Cancer: A Survivor's Guide for When Treatment Ends and the Rest of Your Life Begins, by Marisa Weiss and Ellen Weiss. This book provides plenty of information about how to more forward after treatment.

The Doggone Days of Summer

Summer 2009

Since Mom ends up with an ambiguous BRCA testing result—we both have the same variant of unknown significance—she undergoes a prophylactic mastectomy and has an expander inserted. The lab reports that they've seen the variant in three different families, but it only seems to track with cancer in *one out of three*. However, we are another family to add to their database. I'm no statistician, but to me the odds seem to change to *two out of four*.

~

Only weeks later, I'm at another funeral home. The son of Mom's and Pop's neighbors is being laid to rest after a tragic swimming accident. Ross was a fine young man, recently accepted to a prestigious college. While growing up, he spent hours playing board games and backyard catch with Alex and Nick. The boys cried when I first told them the news. As they sit in their ill-fitting, rarely worn suits, my sons wear solemn, stricken expressions. The pews are filled with mourning family members and friends from scouting, church, and the grocery store where he worked part-time.

We never expect someone so young, with such a bright future, to die.

~

At a follow-up with Rock Star Surgeon, I scrutinize the slight puckering of the scar on my right foob. I touch a tiny bump, no bigger than a grain of rice.

Seasoned Nurse Practitioner, a trim woman with silver hair, comes in the exam room first. Introducing herself as a new member of their practice, she spends a long time going over my medical history and gives me a thorough breast exam. Warm and knowledgeable, she puts me at ease.

"I think what you're feeling is scar tissue," she reassures me. "But we'll get the doctor to take a look."

Moments later, Rock Star Surgeon walks in.

"Nice tie!" I say. *Why do I have such a fixation with his neckwear?*

"Thanks. I like your glasses," he replies, admiring my new tortoiseshell frames. "They make you look intelligent."

"Good. My plan is working!"

"She *is* intelligent!" Seasoned Nurse Practitioner interjects.

"I know she is," he replies.

"We're joking," I explain to her.

"How's your mom?"

"Her last mammogram showed abnormalities in her right breast, and she had the same confusing BRCA results, so she just had a second mastectomy. She still has the expander, but she's doing fine."

"Good to hear." He glances at my chart. "Would you mind opening your gown so I can get a better look at your reconstruction? I don't mean to embarrass you."

"Embarrass me? You're kidding! I lift my shirt whenever I see a white lab coat. I've scared the CVS photo lab guys a few times."

They both laugh.

"I've got to remember that one," says Seasoned Nurse Practitioner.

I unwrap my gown, revealing Dr. L'Artiste's handiwork.

"Wow, you've got great skin!" Rock Star Surgeon says.

Now it's my turn to laugh. Beauty truly *is* in the eyes of the beholder! From the perspective of a breast surgeon, my middle-aged skin drapes nicely over the implants, a softer, more natural result than younger women with taut, firm skin would get.

"What do you think about this?" asks Seasoned Nurse Practitioner, pointing to the questionable spot.

He touches the tiny bump.

"Scar tissue, nothing to worry about," Rock Star Surgeon pronounces, pulling my gown closed. "You got a really nice outcome."

"Thanks. It pays to go with the Dream Team."

He blushes. Now he's the one who's embarrassed.

~

With a new-found commitment to live in the moment, I surprise Ryan with tickets to a Coldplay concert. We enjoy live music, but don't see it often enough. Though the venue is jam-packed, we find a spot on the grassy lawn to spread our blanket.

The band kicks off with their hit song "Yellow" as dozens of fluorescent beach balls sail overhead. As the music soars, the crowd sways to the beat.

The lyrics of the song "Fix You" were supposedly inspired by Gwyneth Paltrow, the lead

Divine Secret: You can find your "new normal."

Life never goes back to how it was before. Some Pink Sisters will deal with constant reminders: long-term or residual effects from surgery, radiation, chemo, or adjuvant drug therapy. Sadly, those with late-stage cancer may face treatment for the rest of their lives. But for many of us, cancer will recede to the shadowy corners of our lives, no longer hogging the spotlight. And, maybe if we look hard enough, we can discover a few silver linings.

singer's wife. *How awesome is that?* She's beautiful, talented, and famous. Not only is she married to Chris Martin, rock superstar, she used to date Ben Affleck and Brad Pitt. She's BFFs with Beyonce and JayZ. Her pal, Stella McCartney, gives her first dibs on designer outfits. Plus, Steven Spielberg's her god-father!

I start to feel this churlish sensation in my gut, like I did around Sunny Survivor. *Oh my goodness! I'm actually jealous of Gwyneth Paltrow!*

But then again, who isn't?

A wave of relief washes over me. *Ah, it's good to feel normal!*

Mesmerized by the songs, my heart floats above the crowd. As the band leaves the stage, Ryan and I hold our cellphones skyward, the contemporary version of waving Bic lighters to request an encore.

Resources: Cancer Memoirs:

Here are some of my favorites:
- *Why I Wore Lipstick to My Mastectomy*, by Geralyn Lucas
- *Bald in the Land of Big Hair*, by Joni Rodgers
- *Nordie's at Noon: The Personal Stories of Four Women "Too Young" For Breast Cancer*, by Patti Balwanz, Kim Carlos, Jennifer Johnson, and Jana Peters
- *Cancer Is a Bitch: I'd Rather Be Having a Midlife Crisis*, by Gail Konop Baker
- *The Middle Place*, by Kelly Corrigan
- *The Foremost Good Fortune*, by Susan Conley

It's a Bird! It's a Plane! It's Anecdote Girl!

Fall 2009

At this point, I've passed my two-year "cancer-versary." Mom has returned to the operating room to swap out her expander for an implant. We both keep moving forward, one foot in front of the other.

But when I hear that Patrick Swayze has died, it's like a punch to my gut. I still struggle with melancholy at times, saddened over the losses of Sandra, Carl, Bill, and Ross, along with so many Pink Sisters. I question why bad things happen to good people. My faith reminds me that I'm "looking through a glass, darkly," but the reflections are cloudy, disproportionate, and confusing. Death can seem cruel and random, nonsensical.

In Alice Sebold's bestseller *The Lovely Bones*, after Susie Salmon, the adolescent narrator, is murdered, she lands in her own special slice of heaven—an idyllic school playground shaded by a large tree. This concept intrigues and inspires me; could the afterlife be personalized for each of us?

If so, I hope Patrick Swayze relocates to an ethereal ranch with an onsite dance studio with mirrored walls and balance barres, where he can spend eternity riding horses and waltzing with his beautiful wife.

As for me, I hope my section of Heaven will be filled with books, chocolate fountains, and cloud-trained puppies. I want to feel the refreshing spray of a waterfall, see majestic mountain views, hear the roar of ocean waves, and savor the aroma of freshly-baked bread. I want to spend eternity with my loved ones; though, for a few of them, I'd be fine with a quick wave from a passing cumulus puff every now and then.

~

One morning, I read a newspaper article that causes me to spill my coffee. The U.S. Preventative Services Task Force (USPSTF) has issued new breast cancer screening guidelines. They now recommend that women don't need routine mammograms until age 50. They've concluded that routine mammograms for women aged 40 to 49 are not cost effective, because 1,904 women would have to be screened to save *one* life. The panel also notes that for every positive finding of cancer, many women undergo biopsies that turn out benign, causing them unnecessary stress and anxiety.

Well, hello! I'm that one out of 1,904!

I was the one diagnosed with invasive breast cancer at age 45 after I was called back following a routine mammogram!

The radiologist who performed my initial diagnostic mammogram told me the lesion was deep inside my breast, in a location where I wouldn't have felt it by self-exam until it had grown much larger.

After multiple sonograms, a stereotactic biopsy, more diagnostic mammograms, and a breast MRI, doctors finally discovered that I had not one, but *two* invasive ductal tumors, along with cellular changes between the malignancies.

Maybe I'm just an anecdote, of statistical insignificance. But I'm also an anomaly with a big mouth, sharing my Adventures in Cancerland. So, I ask: *Which one of you pointy-headed statisticians is going to tell my husband and kids I'm expendable? That it's more cost-effective if I'm pushing up daisies?*

I'm sorry for anyone who's suffered the stress and anxiety of undergoing a biopsy that turns out benign…but not *that* sorry!

Because, despite the statistical odds, I was diagnosed at age 45, with (at that time) no known family history. Thanks to yearly mammograms, which I began at age 40, my cancer was caught at an early stage.

~

Over the next few days, this recommendation sets off a shark-feeding media frenzy, the Internet bloody with arguments from medical experts and the survivor community. The American Cancer Society and Komen for the Cure both stand by their recommendations for starting routine mammograms at age 40. The USPSTF affirms their stance, yet eventually adds a disclaimer that doctors should make screening decisions based on a woman's individual risk factors.

This debate proves again one of my Ta-Ta Secrets: *smart doctors do not always agree.*

But, as I learn more about breast cancer research, I start to understand some troubling facts. Despite the sparkly pink spin of fundraising events, we have not made nearly enough progress in the fight against breast cancer. The death rate—number of women (and men) dying from breast cancer—has not dropped significantly over the past decade.

This seems confusing at first, so let me explain. Early detection gets a lot of upbeat, reassuring media attention. According to the National Breast Cancer Coalition, however, there's been no significant decline in the number of women *initially* diagnosed with advanced breast cancer, who then die of the disease. The NBCC also states that, percentage-wise, not enough of the money spent fighting breast cancer is targeted for researching and treating Stage IV disease.

There's a huge emphasis on the very good survival rates for women with early-stage breast cancer. No doubt, this is wonderful news. With advances in screening technology, tumors are being discovered at earlier and earlier stages.

Of course, all this early screening brings up valid concerns about overtreatment, a "hot topic" in the medical community. *Are we sometimes carpet-bombing small, indolent tumors with aggressive treatments when a "surgical strike" or even "watchful waiting" would be better?*

During my bout with breast cancer, I told my kids that chemo was like using weed killer or a pesticide to remove noxious plants from your garden. Weed killer might be a good option if you have an uncontrollable invasion of poison ivy. *But would you really want to use it for a single dandelion?* We know that exposure to toxic chemicals—even for the greater good of annihilating cancer cells—is harmful to our health.

But if a tumor is found in *your* breast, would you be willing to forego surgery, radiation, or chemo in the hopes it was a slow-growing cancer that wouldn't cut short your life?

Maybe some Pink Sisters would.

But not me. Not just yet.

We need screening tools that provide both *sensitivity* and *specificity*. For example, breast MRIs are very effective at *sensitivity*, picking up tiny irregularities, but need more *specificity*, the accuracy of predicting if an anomaly is malignant or benign.

Hopefully, the next few years will provide breakthroughs in cancer treatment. Right now, genetic assays of tumor cells are helping doctors customize treatment for each patient. Maybe we're starting to see the beginning of a landslide.

Perhaps there will be a major paradigm shift, such as when the radical mastectomy ("Halsted") procedure went out of favor. First performed in 1882, radical mastectomy was the standard of care until

Divine Secret: Participate in the war against cancer in ways both large and small.

Maybe you can become an advocate for breast cancer research, participate in a clinical trial, or join an ongoing study. Perhaps you can help organize fundraisers, bake casseroles, accompany someone to chemo, or mail an encouraging card.

the mid-1970s. For decades, if you were diagnosed with breast cancer, you underwent removal of not only your breast and all lymph nodes under your arm, but also the major and minor muscles behind your breast. Survivors were left significantly disfigured, often with chronic pain and lymphedema. Contrast that to today, when many women benefit from breast-conserving lumpectomies and less drastic mastectomies.

Early detection gets a lot of media attention. But I fervently hope that we see new treatments for advanced breast cancer. Far too many of my Pink Sisters are dying too young and too soon.

We need a cure. And we need it now!

Resource: BreastCancer2020.org

This website, hosted by the National Breast Cancer Coalition, an organization focused on eradicating breast cancer by the year 2020, has issued "Ending Breast Cancer: A Baseline Status Report," packed full of insightful information.

Resource: Wondering when to get a mammogram?

Read for yourself the recommended guidelines and discuss with your doctor.
- American Cancer Society: cancer.org
- Susan G. Komen for the Cure: ww5.komen.org
- USPSTF: uspreventativeservicetaskforce.org

Resource: Important recent books about cancer:

- *The Harm We Do: A Doctor Breaks Rank about Being Sick in America*, by Dr. Otis Brawley, the chief medical and scientific officer of the American Cancer Society
- *The Emperor of All Maladies: A Biography of Cancer*, Dr. Siddhartha Mukherjee's Pulitzer Prize–winning historical account of our understanding of the disease

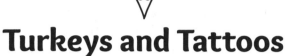

Turkeys and Tattoos

It's been over three years since my diagnosis; breast cancer no longer gobbles up my energy and attention like a gluttonous Ms. Pac-Man. The disease changed me, but does not define me. Yet hearing about the diagnoses of people I know—my former manager, the mom of Nick's friend, a teacher from Larissa's preschool—triggers a visceral, heart-crumpling response.

~

Mom calls to tell me she's finished her last stage of reconstruction. "Joanna, guess what? I'm done. Just got my pigmentation."

I laugh. She's explaining—in a delicate way—that she's had color applied to the skin surrounding her fake nipples to create the appearance of an areola.

"Mom, you got tattoos! Don't hide behind some dainty euphemism. Own it! You have tats!"

Maybe I need a leather jacket and a Harley-Davidson, too."

We both crack up at the mental image of her wearing a skull and crossbones do-rag, straddling a loud motorcycle.

~

Nobody enjoys hanging out at the oncologist's office, but that's where I find myself the Friday after Thanksgiving. The day before, I'd cooked turkey and dressing for Ryan's side of the family. Luckily, nothing burned. Everyone is staying through the weekend, but I'm scheduled for a follow-up with Dr. Point Guard.

The Cancer Center is jam-packed with people. All the chairs are taken in the check-in area, so I stand next to a slender woman with gray hair.

"I can't believe how crowded it is," she remarks. "Who'd think that so many people would want to see their oncologist the day after Thanksgiving?"

"Well, my in-laws are in town," I deadpan. "So I didn't mind."

She doubles over in laughter.

Egged on by her response, I hold out my arms, palm side up, as if I'm balancing scales. "Oncologist or in-laws?" I raise and lower my hands. "In-laws or oncologist?"

She struggles for breath.

People in the chairs nearby look at us, wondering what's so funny.

"Tell them!" she gasps.

I recount our conversation and everyone laughs at the punch line. The story gets repeated again and again, the sweet sound of laugher wafting through the oncology waiting room.

(Disclaimer: my in-laws are wonderful people, but I'll say most anything for a laugh!)

~

Since I have a family history of osteoporosis, combined with my current lack of estrogen, Dr. Point Guard keeps close tabs on my bone health. Several weeks before Christmas, I go to the newly-constructed imaging center for a bone density scan. The test is simple and easy. I dress in yet another ugly hospital gown and recline on a table while the machine takes images.

Afterwards, I dress and the friendly, young technician walks me to the exit. She hands me an envelope.

"What's this?"

"Just a little something for you."

I open the envelope. It's a thank-you note from the hospital! For allowing them to perform my bone density scan.

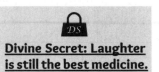

Divine Secret: Laughter is still the best medicine.

Drugs may stop working, cause an allergic reaction, or result in troublesome side effects. But laughter always brings a measure of relief.

"You've got to be kidding." I laugh. Apparently, more health facilities are imbibing the "Service Excellence" kool-aid. "Well, thank *you* for that most excellent scan!"

As I walk by the checkout area, I give the clerks a little wave and shout-out. "Great job, guys. Best bone density scan e-vah!"

61

Getting in the Last Word

Spring 2010

Mom and I attend a luncheon for breast cancer survivors. Hundreds of attendees congregate in a massive hotel ballroom. I wear a new turquoise blouse that fits snugly over the perky new girls, which I'm happy to accentuate, and looser over my midsection, which I'm eager to hide.

We end up sitting at a table with four other Pink Sisters. One woman, newly diagnosed, has come alone, so Mom and I try to offer encouragement as we answer her questions.

As the meal is served, the other three ladies at our table apologize for their reserved demeanor.

"We don't mean to seem unfriendly," a woman wearing a white sweater decorated by pink ribbon embroidery explains, her eyes welling with tears. "We just lost a dear friend."

"I'm so sorry," I say. "I hate this stupid disease."

Mom and Newly Diagnosed Lady echo my sentiments, expressing their sympathy.

"The four of us went through treatment together. It hurts that she's not here."

The trio of ladies dab their eyes and sniffle, their grief visceral.

Our table sits in silence. Sometimes words are so *fricking* inadequate.

Yet over dessert, the keynote speaker makes everyone laugh, telling jokes only a sorority sister can appreciate, such as how the folds of flesh after her skin-sparing mastectomy looked like she was smuggling a Shar-Pei puppy underneath her blouse. The woman at the podium mentions her oncology surgeon by name. *It's Rock Star Surgeon!* The crowd goes wild, as if he's the Justin Bieber for cancer survivors.

The keynote speaker also makes us cry, reminding us that underneath the pink glitter and positive attitudes lurk loss and pain. I look around the ballroom and see so many beautiful women joined in sisterhood, scarred yet undaunted.

~

I attend a pool party hosted by one of the members from the swanky support group. Her home is gorgeous, the pool area and landscaping as plush as you'd find at a spa. Dozens of women mill around, chatting and sampling appetizers, but none of us wear a swimsuit or actually step into the pool.

It's a warm evening, so I'm a bit surprised no one jumps in the cool, refreshing water. Of course, I didn't pack my suit either. *Are we all self-conscious? Worried about messing up our hair?* Maybe we're painfully aware that some are at a point in treatment where donning a swimsuit is too complicated.

Fetching a glass of white wine, I glance around the patio, looking for familiar faces. The crowd at this support group tends to skew young, with many in their 30s and 40s. Everyone looks stylish, with chunky jewelry, cute capris, or sundresses.

I talk with a few women I've met before, who update me on the purchase and renovation of a residential property being designed as a "Pink House." They describe the yoga classes, support groups, and fundraisers envisioned for the new facility.

Working my way through the crowd, I end up as part of a small group chatting with a newcomer, a young, attractive brunette recently diagnosed and facing surgery. I'm drawn to the mischievous twinkle in her eye, her self-effacing humor, and her bling-y "Under Construction" t-shirt. Bubbly Survivor asks me several questions about my experience. As the group leader calls everyone to the covered seating area for the speaker presentation, we're left standing alone.

"Let's go find a spot," I say, turning toward the crowd.

"Wait," she pleads, touching my arm. Suddenly, the sparkle in her eye dims. "I just want to know...do you ever...get to the point where...you don't think about cancer every minute of every day?"

Caught off guard, I hesitate for a second.

"Yes," I answer, trying to soothe the anxiety in her expression. "Yes! Many of us do get to that point." I know she's been diagnosed with DCIS—the earliest, non-invasive stage—and should have an excellent survival rate.

"Really?"

"When you're in the middle of it, the cancer's all-consuming. Your life revolves around doctor appointments and surgical schedules. I know everyone is telling you that your prognosis is very good, which is true. Still, it's scary."

"Definitely."

"Give yourself time to process everything. Going through surgery and reconstruction is a long haul. It's been three years since my diagnosis and it took me a while to find my way back. Most days, I stuff my cancer thoughts into a tiny box and hide it on a dark shelf in my emotional closet. But I do get edgy before follow-up appointments or worried if I have some weird symptom."

She nods, listening intently.

"But I've gotten to the point where I no longer think about cancer every day, every week, or even every month. Sometimes it feels more like a bad dream—unless it's October, when it truly turns into a pink nightmare."

She laughs and gives me a hug. "Thank you."

$\sim$

Weeks later, on our annual family beach vacation, we're exhausted after a fun day of riding bikes, playing in the surf, building sandcastles, and eating crab legs at the seafood buffet. Ryan and the kids are fast asleep.

Yet I toss and turn, unable to stop thinking about Bubbly Survivor and how her sunny, upbeat expression turned into frozen fear. There are so many things I want to tell her. *Accept the foil-covered casseroles. Choose doctors who are both smart and nice. Hand out "Stupid Passes" when needed. Don't feel guilty if you hate the color pink. Reach out to a sorority sister whenever you feel scared or alone.*

But I also think about what is more difficult to say: although her prognosis is very good, some of our Pink Sisters will deal with Stage IV disease every day for the rest of their lives. Over recent years, more and more are able to stop or slow progression, living with cancer much like a chronic disease. Others have tried every promising new drug, cutting-edge treatment, and ground-breaking clinical trial—holding onto hope and exhausting all options—yet their disease spreads, unabated.

Early detection is great, but it's not nearly enough.

I cannot speak for my Stage IV sisters because I have not walked in their shoes.

Instead, I'll share what they have told me. That they have good days and bad days. That they cling tightly to hope against unfavorable odds. That it hurts when people avoid them, as if their cancer were contagious. That the bad days can be difficult and lonely. But when they are able, they try to squeeze every last drop of joy from each good day.

I want to reassure Bubbly Survivor that many of us will finish cancer treatment and move forward in our lives. But I also want her to realize that some will face lingering side effects, such as chronic pain or mental fogginess, reminded of cancer on a daily basis. And to never forget our Stage IV Sisters struggling to live as fully and as long as possible—still waiting and hoping for a cure.

Lastly, I want to reassure her that even in the darkest hours—though the sharp claws of cancer may silence lungs and still hearts—the disease will never, ever break the bonds of love.

Crawling out of bed, I fumble to the desk in the dark, bumping my knee on the dresser. Turning on my laptop, I listen to the soft sounds of my family breathing and begin to type.

Maybe you, or someone you love, just became a member of the "pink sorority" nobody wants to join. Perhaps you noticed a lump while showering or were called back after your mammogram...

Divine Secret: Cancer can do a lot of bad things, but it can never, ever extinguish love.

Acknowledgements

I'm indebted to so many people for sharing their feedback over the years I've worked on this book. Lisa Simone and Lana Hendershott offered an abundance of much-needed red ink. Bethany Aronow and Krysti Hughett provided encouragement when this book was just a shadow of an idea.

Thanks also to Kathleen Adey, Nancy Bowden, and Donna Mathoslah, my very first readers, and founders of Four Blondes Publishing. Along the way, I received helpful suggestions from a number of readers: Betty Vitek, Laura Spinella, Jeannine Jamieson, Lisa Thornton, Jennifer Poole, Karen Shayne, Barbara Claypole White, Anne Woodman, Carole Sanek, Lisa Grey, Kim Selig, Jennifer Haag, Wayne Drumheller, Mary Carson, Gail Moore. Thanks also to my fellow students (and instructor) in Jennifer McGaha's spring 2012 memoir writing class.

Sending love and appreciation to my circle of friends and family, who have supported me every step of the way.

Thanks also to the South Carolina Writers' Workshop, where my first chapter won their nonfiction contest several years ago, spurring my confidence to move forward.

Thanks also to some special teachers who encouraged my love of reading and writing: the late Jewel Wimbish, third-grade teacher extraordinaire; Dr. Jerome Loving, professor of English at Texas A&M; and the late Rita Gallagher, a gifted instructor and classy lady. I have been fortunate to surround myself with a talented team of people. Thanks to Sarah Holroyd for editing and book interior design, to Sarah Jensen for the book cover, and to Betsy Thorpe for providing astute answers to all my questions. Thanks also to Marc Silver, Joni Rodgers, Jennifer Johnson, Mindy Greenstein, Melissa Ackerman, Jennifer Smith, and Debbie Cantwell for their kind words of praise.

Any errors are mine, and probably the result of my not listening to someone's good advice.

About the Author

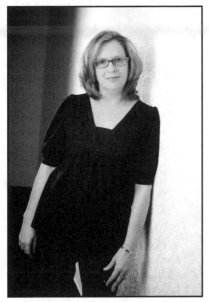

Photo © Glenn Roberson Photography

Although she doesn't plan on relocating there any time in the near future, Joanna Chapman hopes Heaven will have comfy chairs for reading, free wi-fi, and complimentary mimosas.

Joanna lives near a large Southern city with her supportive but cranky husband, three beloved yet hard-headed children, and two sweet but crazy dogs. A graduate of Texas A&M University, she has worked as a corporate trainer, college instructor, and stay-at-home mom.

Divine Secrets of the Ta-Ta Sisterhood: Pledging the Pink Sorority is her first book.

Joanna would love to hear from readers. To contact her, send an e-mail to her publisher, Cosmic Casserole Press, at cosmiccasserole@gmail.com.